EAT SO WHAT!

THE SCIENCE OF FAT-SOLUBLE VITAMINS

EVERYTHING YOU NEED TO KNOW ABOUT VITAMINS A, D, E AND K

LA FONCEUR

CONTENTS

Contents

INTRODUCTION

The term "vitamin" is often thrown around. While we may have some knowledge regarding vitamins, do we really know all about vitamins? While we may have some vitamin knowledge, our awareness is often limited to what we hear from health advocates or simply dietary supplement manufacturing companies. You may come across countless articles promoting the benefits of vitamins, and they often conclude with recommendations for specific supplements.

The aim of scientific discoveries is not to substitute natural food with artificial or genetically modified food. Instead, the goal is to comprehend what is necessary for a healthy and ailment-free life and modify our lifestyle and dietary habits accordingly. However, rather than making these changes, we often opt for shortcuts and rely on supplements. This is mainly due to the influence of advertising and the pharmaceutical industry. Nowadays, you can find supplements for almost everything on the market.

Supplements have become easily accessible and convenient, saving time and effort. Many rely on supplements due to a busy lifestyle and limited knowledge about what their body needs for optimal health. This dependence may stem from fear or a reluctance to put in the effort to obtain necessary nutrients.

There are many misleading approaches available in the market. It is important to have accurate information because half-baked knowledge can be more harmful than no knowledge at all. For instance, suppose you read an article about the importance of a particular nutrient for health and the diseases caused by its deficiency. With this, you have become aware of the importance of getting this nutrient. But, if you see an advertisement for a supplement that claims to provide this nutrient, you may be tempted to take it without knowing the daily recommended amount for your age or its side effects, even though this nutrient can be easily taken from natural sources. Although supplements may be beneficial, they are not regulated by the FDA, and overdose is common and dangerous. Unless your doctor has prescribed a supplement for a medical condition or deficiency, it is best to rely on whole foods to meet your nutrient needs.

When questioned about the benefits of fat-soluble vitamins, the usual response from most individuals would be vitamin A for vision, vitamin D for bone health, vitamin K for healing wounds, and vitamin E for skin and blood thinning. However, these vitamins do much more than that. Consuming them through natural sources can provide various other health benefits that may surprise you. In fact, these vitamins have been known to affect your health in numerous ways, some of which are yet to be fully discovered. This is why relying on vitamin supplements may not provide the same results that can be effortlessly obtained through natural sources. If you're not focusing on getting your necessary vitamins from food, you're missing out on a lot of potential health benefits.

Get all your answers about fat-soluble vitamins A, D, E, and K with the ***Eat So What! Science of Fat-Soluble Vitamins*** book. Learn about their crucial role in maintaining good health and the latest scientific findings and how these can affect your vitamin decisions. Find out about other vitamins you may not know of and whether or not you should take them. Clear up common vitamin-related dilemmas, such as how to tell if you're deficient in vitamins and when to get tested.

Learn about the advantages of combining specific vitamins for optimal health benefits, as well as the potential consequences of taking certain vitamins with particular foods or medications. This guide covers both beneficial and harmful combinations of vitamins, as well as the advantages and drawbacks of fortified foods and vitamin supplements.

Furthermore, learn about nutrient-rich vegetarian options that are high in vitamins A, D, E, and K. By consuming these foods, you can avoid vitamin deficiencies and maintain good overall health, reducing the likelihood of infections and chronic illnesses such as cancer, diabetes, high blood pressure, and cognitive decline. Plus, explore some nutritious and easy-to-cook vegetarian recipes that can be included in your diet to maximize the health benefits of vitamins A, D, E, and K.

UNIT 1

BASICS OF VITAMINS

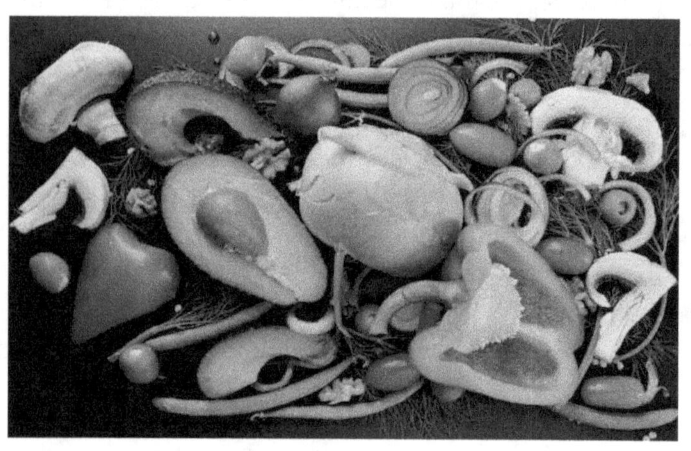

Chapter 1

BASICS OF VITAMINS

Vitamins are organic compounds required by the body in small quantities to perform various normal functions Vitamins can be essential or non-essential. Essential nutrients are crucial for the normal function of the body, and the body cannot produce them, so they must be obtained through food.

Vitamins differ from macronutrients such as carbohydrates, proteins, and fats because they do not provide energy and are required in smaller quantities. They are called micronutrients because they are needed in small amounts, but this does not make them any less important than macronutrients.

While vitamins are now a topic of general discussion, it may surprise you that they were discovered not so long ago. In fact, all known vitamins were identified during the period between 1912 and 1948.

ESSENTIAL NUTRIENTS

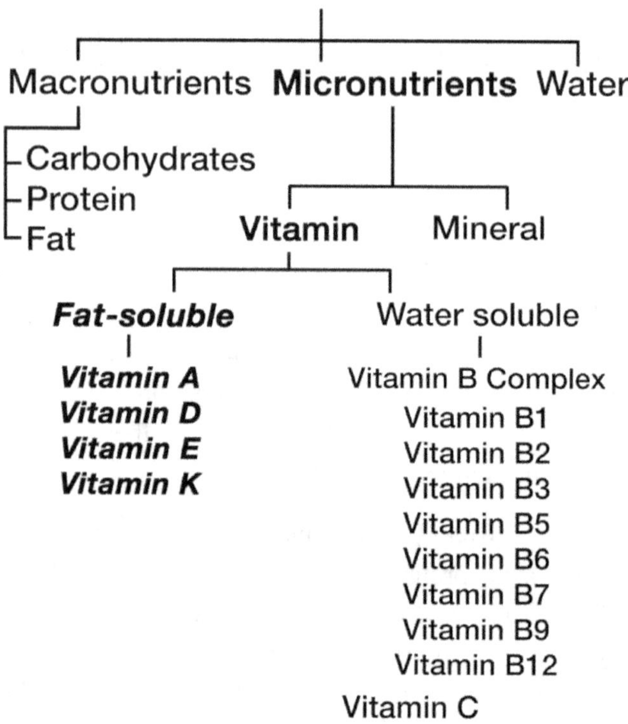

CLASSIFICATION OF ESSENTIAL VITAMINS

There are 13 essential vitamins that are classified as water-soluble vitamins and fat-soluble vitamins.

Water-Soluble Vitamins

Water-soluble Vitamins are Vitamin B1, B2, B3, B4, B5, B6, B7, B12 and Vitamin C. These vitamins are called water-soluble as they dissolve in water. There are nine of them, including Vitamin B1 to B12 and Vitamin C. Since they dissolve in water, they are easily absorbed, and any excess is excreted in urine quickly without being stored in the body. This is why it is essential to consume water-soluble vitamins regularly to maintain adequate levels.

Fat-Soluble Vitamins

Fat-soluble vitamins are Vitamin A, Vitamin D, Vitamin E and Vitamin K. Fat-soluble vitamins are not soluble in water but instead, dissolve in fats. There are five vitamins that are classified as fat-soluble vitamins - vitamins A, D, E, and K, and these are absorbed by the body in a similar way to dietary fats. When you consume fat-soluble vitamins with healthy fats, their absorption in the intestine increases. Unlike water-soluble vitamins, fat-soluble vitamins are stored in the body and can be used whenever the body requires them. The body stores fat-soluble vitamins in the liver, muscles, and fatty tissue (adipocytes). This means that a continuous supply of fat-soluble vitamins is not necessary, as they are not excreted from the body as quickly as water-soluble vitamins. However, consuming adequate amounts is important to reach the daily recommended intake.

Too much of these vitamins can lead to toxicity (Hypervitaminosis), especially for vitamin A from animal sources (retinol) and vitamin D. Toxicity usually occurs when taking supplements, not from food. A balanced diet typically provides sufficient amounts of fat-soluble vitamins. The following chapters will discuss these five vitamins (A, D, E, and K) in detail.

Why do I need fat-soluble vitamins?

Your body requires fat-soluble vitamins to carry out vital physiological processes. In their absence, your body becomes weak and vulnerable to infections and chronic diseases. These vitamins are essential for building your immune system and protecting you from diseases, strengthening your bones, boosting your cognitive health, and reducing the risk of cardiovascular diseases. Overall, fat-soluble vitamins are crucial in maintaining your overall well-being and happiness.

What if I am deficient in fat-soluble vitamins?

Each fat-soluble vitamin plays a unique role in the body. For example, a lack of vitamin A can lead to night blindness, vitamin D deficiency can cause osteomalacia, vitamin E deficiency can result in oxidative stress, and vitamin K deficiency can cause hemorrhage.

Which vitamin deficiency is most common?

Surprisingly, vitamin D deficiency is currently one of the most common vitamin deficiencies worldwide and has become a global concern with serious health consequences. This deficiency is a reflection of our lifestyle and indiscipline. Although out-of-control risk factors such as aging and malabsorption syndromes cannot be controlled, other undisciplined lifestyle choices such as sedentariness, lack of sunlight, and obesity as well as poor food choices can be easily acted upon and successfully prevent Vitamin D deficiency.

Types of Vitamin Deficiency

There are two types of vitamin deficiency:

Primary deficiency

Secondary deficiency

Primary deficiency

Primary deficiency can happen when you do not eat enough foods that are high in vitamins.

Reasons:

- Poor diet.
- Unavailability of a particular vitamin-rich food in that region.

Secondary deficiency

A secondary deficiency can happen when the body cannot properly absorb or use vitamins.

Reasons:

- Poor lifestyle choices such as smoking and drinking alcohol.
- Use of medications that interfere with the absorption of vitamins.
- An underlying disorder that limits the absorption of vitamins.

Are vitamins antioxidants?

Let's first understand what are antioxidants:

Oxidative Stress and Antioxidants

Oxidative processes are normal in the body and are important to provide energy for many cellular functions. Oxygen is used by cells to generate energy, with free radicals being produced as a by-product. In small amounts, free radicals are beneficial as they can kill pathogens and regulate cell growth and death. However, excessive free radicals can cause chronic diseases. The body produces free radicals during normal cell metabolism, but external sources like radiation, pollution, cigarette smoke, and medication can also expose you to these harmful free radicals. Drinking alcohol and consuming excess sugar, and fat may also contribute to free radical production.

Free radicals are unpaired electrons that like to be paired. Antioxidants are produced by the body to balance free radicals and stop them from causing damage. Oxidative stress occurs when there is an imbalance between free radicals and antioxidants, and the accumulation of free radicals in the body cannot be gradually eliminated. This process causes unpaired free radicals to pair with electrons in fat tissue, proteins, and DNA, and this can damage cells and tissues, increasing the risk of developing chronic and degenerative diseases like cancer, rheumatoid arthritis, cataracts, diabetes, aging, as well as cardiovascular and neurodegenerative diseases.

Some foods have antioxidant properties and can delay or inhibit cellular damage by their free radical scavenging ability. These antioxidant foods are capable of breaking the free radical chain reaction by donating an electron to a free radical without destabilizing themselves. The three vitamins that act as antioxidants are pro-vitamin A (carotenoids), vitamin E, and vitamin C. Since these micronutrients cannot be produced by the body, they must be obtained through the diet.

Recent research indicates that other vitamins such as Vitamin K, Vitamin D, niacin, pyridoxine, and riboflavin, in addition to antioxidant vitamins A, C, and E, exhibit antioxidant properties and have the potential to manage and prevent diseases. However, further studies are necessary to determine their exact role as antioxidants.

Plant-Based Antioxidants

Nutrient

Vitamins: Vitamin A, Vitamin C and Vitamin E.

Minerals: Copper, zinc, selenium, and manganese.

Non-nutrient

Phytochemicals: Polyphenols such as flavonoids, lignans, and stilbenes.

Are vitamins Anti-inflammatory?

Let's first understand what is inflammation

Is inflammation good or bad?

Both. The process of inflammation is a natural defense mechanism of the body. It is the process by which the immune system identifies and eliminates harmful and foreign bodies, and begins the healing process. there are two types of inflammation, acute inflammation, which lasts for a few days, is helpful in cases where the body experiences injury or harm. For instance, if you have a cut on your finger, your body sends inflammatory cells to the injury site to start the healing process.

Chronic inflammation is a type of inflammation that occurs over a longer period of time and can last for several months or even years. Even when there is no external threat, your body continues to send inflammatory cells, which can create an ongoing and unnecessary inflammatory condition. This can eventually harm healthy tissues in the long run. Chronic inflammation is the primary cause of many chronic diseases, including rheumatoid arthritis, chronic obstructive pulmonary disease (COPD), diabetes, and cancer.

Chronic inflammation can be caused by several factors, including environmental pollutants, auto-immune diseases, infection, and untreated acute inflammation. Lifestyle factors, such as stress, obesity, alcohol consumption, and smoking, can also contribute to inflammation in the body. It is crucial to treat inflammation promptly, as not doing so can result in life-threatening consequences.

All fat-soluble vitamins A, D, E, and K are anti-inflammatory. Each one has a different pathway to reduce inflammation in the body, which will be discussed in detail in their respective chapters.

NON-ESSENTIAL VITAMINS

Non-essential vitamins are the vitamins that the body can make. Most vitamins are essential and cannot be produced by the body, except for vitamins D, K, and B7.

• The skin produces Vitamin D when exposed to certain UVB rays from direct sunlight.

• Vitamin K2 is produced in the intestines, but not in sufficient amounts, so a diet rich in vitamin K is still necessary to meet the daily recommended intake.

• Biotin or B7 cannot be synthesized by the body but can be produced by intestinal flora.

Although technically non-essential, these vitamins are still considered essential nutrients because they play a crucial role in the normal growth and development of the body.

NON-NUTRIENTS

Certain substances found in food do not provide any calories but may have positive effects on human health. These substances are known as non-nutrients and include fiber, water, and phytochemicals like flavonoids, curcumin, and polyphenols. While early studies suggest that non-nutrients can improve overall health, more research is needed to classify them as nutrients officially.

Some Interesting Facts About Fat-Soluble Vitamins

• Vitamins were discovered and identified between the years 1912 and 1948.

• The fresher the fruits and vegetables, the more vitamins they will contain.

• Different vitamins react differently to heat. Cooking may increase or decrease the vitamin content of the food.

• While Vitamins D and K are classified as essential nutrients, your body has the ability to produce them.

• Even though the sun rises every day, vitamin D deficiency remains one of the most prevalent nutrient deficiencies worldwide.

• Consuming fat-soluble vitamins in the morning on an empty stomach does not provide much benefit.

Chapter 2

NOT TRUE VITAMINS BUT STILL VITAMINS!

Are there any vitamins other than the 13 already known?

Some compounds were previously classified as vitamins but were later either renamed to already identified vitamins or removed from the list because their health effects were not proven enough to be considered true vitamins. These vitamins that are no longer vitamins still have some positive impact on health. These include:

Vitamin F: Vitamin F was reclassified as essential fatty acids which are comprised of — alpha-linolenic acid (ALA) - omega-3 fatty acids and linoleic acid (LA) - omega-6 fatty acids. These essential fatty acids are required in large amounts, so it does not fit the true definition of a vitamin and has therefore been removed from the vitamin category.

Vitamin G: Vitamin G or riboflavin was reclassified as Vitamin B2.

Vitamin H: Vitamin H was reclassified as Vitamin B7 or biotin.

Vitamin J: Vitamin J or flavin was similar to vitamin G and was reclassified as Vitamin B2.

Vitamin L1: Vitamin L1 or anthranilic acid, an amino acid, was once considered a vitamin but later proved to be non-essential to human health.

Vitamin M: Vitamin M is also known as folate (in some countries as folic acid) or vitamin B11. Green leafy vegetables, soybeans, and oranges are good sources of vitamin M.

Vitamin PP: Vitamin Pellagra-Prevention or vitamin PP was reclassified as vitamin B3.

Vitamin T: Vitamin T is also known as torutilin, or Factor T. It may increase stamina and improve white and red blood cell function. Some good examples of foods rich in vitamin T are yeast, sesame seeds, and fungi.

Vitamin U: Vitamin U is a compound found in raw cabbage juice that was previously used to heal gut ulcers. Hence the name vitamin U. Vitamin U can heal stomach ulcers and reduce cholesterol levels. Some good examples of foods rich in vitamin U are cabbage, kale, celery, spinach, and beetroot.

Chapter 3

FOOD FORTIFCATION

What is food fortification?

Food fortification and food enrichment sound similar but are different. Both involve adding essential nutrients such as vitamins and minerals to food and share the common goal of preventing nutritional deficiencies and promoting public health while minimizing potential health risks. However, food enrichment adds back essential nutrients lost during processing, while fortification adds additional essential nutrients that may not be present or only present in small amounts prior to processing.

Types of Fortifications

Mandatory Fortification is when governments legally oblige food manufacturers to add certain vitamins or minerals, or both, to specified foods. Common examples of mandatory fortifications are the addition of iodine in salt, vitamins—riboflavin, thiamin, and niacin to flour, and vitamins A and D to milk.

Voluntary Fortification allows food producers to add vitamins or minerals, or both, to foods, as long as they comply with the regulatory guidelines of the country. Common examples of voluntary fortifications are breakfast cereal and soy milk.

Are these added micronutrients natural?

These added micronutrients are either derived from plants or animals, or they are synthetic, artificial chemicals created in a laboratory. Food manufacturers add these chemicals to their products during production which contain vitamins and minerals.

How are fortified foods different from dietary supplements?

A dietary supplement is any product that supplements the diet. It can come in the form of a concentrate, extract, metabolite, or combination and may contain vitamins, minerals, amino acids, herbs, or other botanical substances. However, unlike drugs, the effectiveness and safety of supplements are not tested.

Fortified foods and dietary supplements both strive to enhance the nutrition of individuals. Fortified foods contain a mild vitamins and minerals, while supplements utilize concentrated nutrients. Fortification aims to boost the nutritional value of individuals, while supplementation works to rectify any nutritional deficiencies in a person.

Why is food fortification necessary when all the essential nutrients are available through natural food sources?

Fortification is necessary due to poor diet, insufficient essential nutrients in the diet, and the unavailability of certain foods in some areas of the world. Iodized salt is the most crucial and effective fortification for preventing goiter.

Another reason for fortification is the extensive processed food available in the market. This processing is done to enhance the taste and increase the shelf life of the product, but it results in the loss of vital vitamins and minerals. The fortification of food ensures that these lost nutrients are added back to the food.

In order to avoid relying on fortified foods or supplements, it is important to have knowledge of which foods contain specific nutrients, the recommended daily intake of each nutrient, and the ideal combination of foods to achieve optimal nutrition.

Who benefits most from food fortification?

Elderly people and pregnant women have higher nutritional needs. Therefore, fortified foods can meet their increased nutritional demands. Fortified foods are also beneficial for people who have certain food allergies or who follow restricted diets.

How do I know if a food is fortified or not?

Always check the nutrition label of your packaged foods. This label will provide details about any added nutrients. If the label specifies that certain essential nutrients have been added, then that food has been fortified.

Is it safe to consume fortified food?

It is generally safe to consume fortified foods, but it is important to note that they should not be relied upon as the sole source of nutrients. Fortification is meant to provide micronutrients that are typically found in a well-balanced diet. While fortified foods may contain higher levels of certain micronutrients, they cannot replace a healthy diet that includes sufficient carbohydrates, protein, essential fats, and other nutrients for optimal health.

Consuming a variety of fortified foods throughout the day can even lead to nutrient overdoses, particularly in children. Many fortified foods available in the market contain levels of vitamins that are not appropriate for children, which can be potentially dangerous.

Is fortified food good or bad?

The food industry often markets highly processed and sugary items as " fortified with essential nutrients," leading people to believe they are making healthy choices. However, these foods are often high in salt, trans fats, saturated fats, and sugar. Simply fortifying a food item does not necessarily make it healthy or beneficial for your health. While micronutrient intake is crucial, healthy food should not just offer essential nutrients but also be low in sugar, salt, trans fats, and saturated fats.

While fortified foods can certainly be included in a healthy diet, they are not sufficient by themselves. You cannot rely on fortified foods to get all the nutrients you need. Your body still needs a complete diet that is rich in fruits and vegetables of different colors along with whole foods to keep you strong and healthy.

UNIT 2

FAT SOLUBLE VITAMINS –

VITMAIN A

VITAMIN D

VITAMIN E

VITAMIN K

Chapter 1

27

VITAMIN A

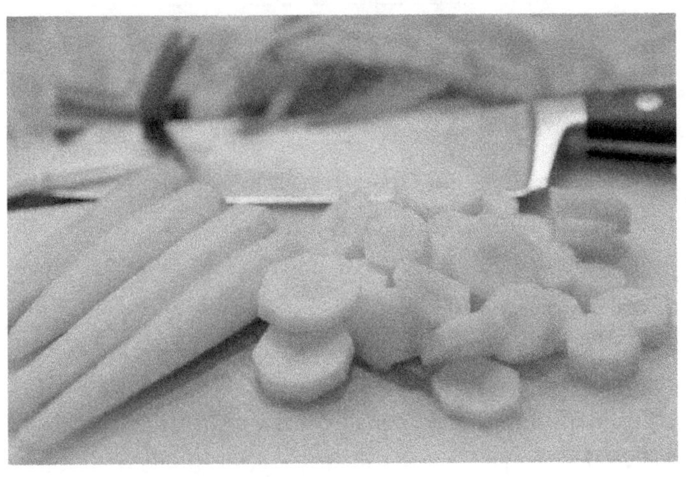

1.

EVERYTHING YOU NEED TO KNOW ABOUT VITAMIN A

Vitamin A, also known as retinol, is an essential fat-soluble vitamin found in both plant-based foods and animal-sourced products. It plays a vital function in growth and development, reproduction, immune function, and eye health. Vitamin A plays a vital role in the growth and differentiation of cells, contributing significantly to the proper development and maintenance of vital organs like the heart, eyes, lungs, and other organs.

What are carotenoids?

Fruits and vegetables get their bright yellow, orange, and red colors from pigments called carotenoids. Some examples of produce containing carotenoids include mangoes, papayas, bell peppers, carrots, and tomatoes. The most common types of carotenoids are beta-carotene, alpha-carotene, beta-cryptoxanthin, lutein, lycopene, and zeaxanthin.

How are carotenoids related to Vitamin A?

Your body has the ability to convert certain carotenoids into Vitamin A. Some examples of these carotenes include beta-carotene, alpha-carotene, and beta-cryptoxanthin.

Types of Vitamin A

Preformed Vitamin A (Animal-based Vitamin A)

As the name suggests, this type of Vitamin A is already made and found in animal products. Preformed Vitamin A (retinol and retinyl esters) is found in dairy products, fortified foods, and vitamin supplements (as retinyl palmitate or retinyl acetate).

Provitamin A Carotenoids (Plant-based Vitamin A)

Provitamin A carotenoids or precursors to Vitamin A are naturally present in fruits and vegetables. Your body converts Provitamin A carotenoids into Vitamin A in your intestine. Beta-carotene is the most common Provitamin A carotenoid present in foods and vitamin supplements.

Non-Provitamin A Carotenoids: Other carotenoids present in food, such as lycopene, lutein, and zeaxanthin, are non-Provitamin A carotenoids and are not converted to Vitamin A in the body but have other vital functions in the body.

How much Vitamin A do I need in a day?

The amount of Vitamin A in food is measured in micrograms (µg) of retinol activity equivalents (RAE). To fulfill the Vitamin A needs of healthy people, the recommended daily intake is:

Age	RDAs for Vitamin A (mcg RAE)	
	Male	Female
0 to 12 months*	400 mcg RAE	400 mcg RAE
1–8 years	300 mcg RAE	300 mcg RAE
9–13 years	600 mcg RAE	600 mcg RAE
14–50+ years	900 mcg RAE	700 mcg RAE

*Adequate Intake (AI)

Adequate intake is the level considered to ensure nutritional adequacy when there is insufficient evidence to develop Recommended Dietary Allowances.

1 mcg RAE is = 1 mcg retinol = 12 mcg dietary beta-carotene = 24 mcg dietary alpha-carotene or beta-cryptoxanthin

Vitamin A doesn't need to be consumed daily. Your body stores extra Vitamin A for future use, meaning if you consume 2-3 mangoes a day, your body will convert beta carotene into Vitamin A and use up the daily required amount while storing the rest for later. Vitamin A is stored in your liver in the form of retinyl esters, like retinyl palmitate. Preformed Vitamin A, or retinyl ester, is converted into retinol after absorption in the lumen, and Provitamin A carotenoids are converted to retinol after absorption. In your body, retinol is oxidized into retinal and retinoic acid, the two main active metabolites of Vitamin A.

Is Provitamin A better than Preformed Vitamin A?

Preformed Vitamin A is better absorbed by the body than beta-carotene but is toxic at high levels. This is more common with preformed Vitamin A supplements and requires monitoring of intake levels. Another drawback is that too much preformed Vitamin A can interfere with the beneficial actions of vitamin D. Also, high levels of it may increase the risk of bone loss, hip fractures, or certain birth defects.

On the other hand, there is no such problem with beta-carotene. Your body can make as much Vitamin A as it needs from beta-carotene, and consuming high levels of beta-carotene is not toxic, so there is no need to monitor intake levels. Although consuming excessive amounts of beta-carotene can cause the skin to turn yellow-orange, this condition is harmless and goes away when you consume less of it. Additionally, beta-carotene acts as an antioxidant and has various positive effects on overall health. Beta carotene may offer you protection against various chronic diseases. Therefore, it is more beneficial to take Vitamin A in the form of beta-carotene.

But too much of anything is not good for health, so consume beta carotene in moderation and get it through food, not dietary supplements. Avoid higher-dose beta-carotene supplements as they may do more harm than good. People with hypothyroidism cannot convert beta-carotene into Vitamin A effectively, and this can be a problem. Studies have also shown that people who smoke or are exposed to asbestos and take beta-carotene supplements of high-dose may have a higher risk of lung cancer and death. So, keep in mind moderation is the key to health.

Does cooking affect the amount of Vitamin A in food?

The body can absorb preformed Vitamin A better than beta carotene. Preformed Vitamin A in the form of retinol can get absorbed about 75% to 100% in the body, and approximately 10% to 30% of beta-carotene from foods are absorbed in the body, but beta-carotene has other important function, such as killing the free radicals in the body. So, despite a low absorption rate, keeping your diet full of beta carotene can have various yet to be discovered health benefits. One way to increase the absorption of beta-carotene from foods is to cook them. Cooking helps release more beta-carotene from food, but it is most effective when you are roasting or baking the food. Boiling for long or stir-frying may result in a 10-15% loss of beta carotene. So, make sure not to boil the food for long or in lots of water to prevent the leaching of beta-carotene in water.

Another way to increase beta-carotene absorption in your body is to cook beta-carotene foods in oil or eat them with other healthy fats, as Vitamin A is a fat-soluble vitamin, and it needs the presence of fat in the body to get properly absorbed.

Is it dangerous to be low in Vitamin A?

Vitamin A is an essential vitamin that your body needs to function properly, and you must get it from food. If you are low in Vitamin A, it can affect many organs, such as the eyes, skin, heart, and reproductive organs. It also affects the defense system of your body against illness. Long-term Vitamin A deficiency can even lead to blindness.

What can happen if I have a Vitamin A deficiency?

Vitamin A deficiency or hypovitaminosis A can be the cause of several disorders. If you are deficient in Vitamin A, you are predisposed to the following conditions:

Eye Problems: Your eyes depend on vitamin A for many vital functions. Vitamin A deficiency can affect overall eye health. The early sign of vitamin A deficiency is difficulty seeing in low light, also known as night blindness. If this deficiency persists over a long period, a person may develop xerophthalmia, a condition where the cells in the cornea change, causing corneal ulcers, lesions, and eventually blindness.

Prone to Infections: Vitamin A is an essential vitamin for your immune system. It helps enhance immune function and plays a crucial role in the development of the immune system and immune responses. Vitamin A regulates the differentiation of immune cells that are necessary for immune tolerance throughout adult life. If you lack Vitamin A, it can impair the function of neutrophils, macrophages, natural killer cells, and T-cell mediated antibody responses, leading to decreased protective mechanisms. Additionally, a deficiency in Vitamin A can reduce mucus production, which increases the risk of invasive pathogens. Vitamin A has therapeutic effects on various infectious digestive diseases, particularly in children, such as diarrhea and hand, foot, and mouth disease.

Infertility: Sufficient intake of Vitamin A is vital for reproduction in both men and women, as well as for several processes during the development of the fetus. Insufficient Vitamin A intake can make it more challenging to get pregnant and result in infertility.

Retard Growth in Children: Vitamin A is essential for growth and development. For children, adequate Vitamin A status is more critical. Vitamin A deficiency contributes to retarded growth in children with persistent diarrhea.

Skin Problems: Vitamin A is essential for reducing inflammation and maintaining healthy skin. If your body lacks Vitamin A, you may be more prone to experiencing skin issues such as eczema and acne.

Additionally, a deficiency in Vitamin A can result in hyperkeratosis, a skin condition where the outer layer of your skin, composed of keratin, becomes thicker than normal.

Respiratory Diseases: Not getting enough Vitamin A can increase your risk of chronic respiratory diseases like chronic obstructive pulmonary disease, pulmonary fibrosis, emphysema, and lung cancer. It can also make you more vulnerable to asthma due to higher susceptibility to oxidative stress. In young children under five years old, low Vitamin A levels are strongly linked to respiratory diseases. Babies and toddlers who lack Vitamin A are at a higher risk of severe respiratory infections like pneumonia, childhood asthma, and measles.

Thyroid Dysfunction: Severe Vitamin A deficiency is associated with a higher risk of goiter and high concentrations of circulating thyroid stimulating hormone (TSH) and thyroid hormones. Vitamin A deficiency interferes with the pituitary thyroid axis. Lack of enough Vitamin A in the body can lead to increased production and secretion of thyroid-stimulating hormone (TSH) by the pituitary gland. It also increases the size of the thyroid gland and reduces iodine uptake by the thyroid gland. Iodine deficiency often co-exists with Vitamin A deficiency. Concurrent iodine deficiency and Vitamin A deficiency produce more severe primary hypothyroidism than iodine deficiency alone.

Anemia: Anemia is a global health issue that can be caused by various factors, including a lack of Vitamin A. Vitamin A helps the body use iron more effectively. It also influences the growth and development of red blood cells and supports iron absorption by forming a complex with nonheme iron. Insufficient Vitamin A intake can lead to abnormal red blood cell shapes, causing microcytic or hypochromic anemia. This type of anemia is characterized by smaller than usual red blood cells (microcytic) with reduced red color (hypochromic) and increased iron storage in the liver. Vitamin A deficiency also reduces the transportation of iron in the body. Treating this type of anemia with iron supplements is ineffective, so Vitamin A supplements are necessary.

Also read: 10 Power Foods to Prevent Anemia in the Book Eat So What! The Power of Vegetarianism.

Weaker Bones: Vitamin A deficiency increases the risk of fractures. Adequate Vitamin A intake (900 mcg for men and 700 mcg for women) is essential for building strong and healthy bones. Vitamin A influences both osteoblasts (bone-building cells) and osteoclasts (bone-breaking down cells). Provitamin A (beta-carotene and beta-cryptoxanthin) protects bones. However, high Vitamin A levels, especially in conjunction with vitamin D deficiency, have been associated with decreased bone density and increased fractures.

What are the causes of Vitamin A deficiency?

There can be various factors that can cause Vitamin A deficiency. The most common reason is due to poor diet, but other factors like disease conditions can also lead to Vitamin A deficiency. Let's see the reasons one by one:

Poor Diet: A diet that lacks Vitamin A-rich foods or inadequate intake of Vitamin A required for physiological needs can cause Vitamin A deficiency in the body.

Fat Malabsorption: Fat malabsorption is a disorder in which your body is unable to absorb fat from your diet. This disorder can be caused by disruptions in your digestion process, including bacterial infection, inadequate digestive enzymes, or faster bowel movements than normal. As Vitamin A is a fat-soluble vitamin, fat malabsorption can affect the absorption of Vitamin A in your body, which can result in Vitamin A deficiency despite consuming a diet rich in Vitamin A.

Certain Disease Conditions: Certain disease conditions, such as impaired pancreatic or biliary secretion, as well as inflammatory bowel diseases like celiac disease and Crohn's disease, can also cause fat malabsorption and hinder Vitamin A absorption in the body, leading to a deficiency of this important nutrient.

Zinc Deficiency: Zinc is crucial for transporting vitamin A in the body. If your diet lacks zinc, it won't impact the absorption or transportation of Vitamin A to the liver. However, it will restrict your body's ability to transfer

Vitamin A from the liver to the body tissues. This may result in Vitamin A deficiency.

Iron Deficiency: Iron deficiency can cause Vitamin A to accumulate in the liver, resulting in reduced plasma retinol concentrations. This can negatively affect the mobilization of Vitamin A from the liver and ultimately decrease plasma retinol concentration, depriving you of the health benefits of Vitamin A.

How do I know if I am deficient in Vitamin A?

The symptoms of Vitamin A deficiency are as follows:

Night Blindness: One of the early indicators of vitamin A deficiency is night blindness, which is when you experience difficulty seeing in low-light conditions but have normal vision in well-lit areas.

Hazy Vision: Another symptom is hazy vision, which is caused by the buildup of keratin in the eyes, known as Bitot's spots. This occurs due to a lack of Vitamin A in the body.

Skin Diseases: If you're experiencing skin problems, you may want to consider whether you're getting enough Vitamin A in your diet. Vitamin A is essential for repairing skin cells. When your body doesn't have enough of this Vitamin, your skin can become dry, scaly, and inflamed, leading to conditions like eczema and acne.

Respiratory Infections: Vitamin A is important for a healthy immune system, and a deficiency in this Vitamin can make you more susceptible to respiratory infections in your chest and throat.

Infertility: Maintaining adequate levels of Vitamin A is crucial for the proper functioning of both male and female reproductive systems. A deficiency in vitamin A can lead to difficulties in conceiving and infertility.

Delayed Growth: Insufficient intake of Vitamin A can result in slow growth or delayed bone growth, leading to stunted growth in children.

Poor Wound Healing: Vitamin A plays a vital role in enhancing the production of collagen type I and fibronectin, which can increase the rate of wound closure and restore the skin structure. If you have low levels of Vitamin A, wounds may not heal properly after injury or surgery.

What should I do if I have Vitamin A deficiency symptoms?

You should consult your doctor if you experience symptoms of Vitamin A deficiency. Your doctor will conclude by examining your history and physical examination and may ask for a serum retinol test if necessary.

Vitamin A Diagnostic Test

A serum retinol blood test is used to measure the amount of Vitamin A in your blood.

A blood sample is taken from your vein on an empty stomach. Alcohol should not be consumed for 24 hours before sample collection.

The healthy range for adults is 20 to 80 mcg/dL. If your reading is less than 20 mcg/dL, you are Vitamin A deficient. However, this test is not accurate because your body stores large amounts of Vitamin A in the liver, so your blood Vitamin A levels will not decrease until your liver stores of Vitamin A are depleted.

The gold standard to assess the overall Vitamin A levels in the body is by measuring the concentration of retinol in the liver through a biopsy. Liver biopsies pose significant risks, so they are not commonly used to assess Vitamin A levels.

If you have a Vitamin A deficiency, your healthcare provider may prescribe high doses of a Vitamin A supplement for a few days. Once your symptoms begin to improve, they will likely switch you to a lower dose of Vitamin A.

If your retinol level is above 30 mcg/dL, taking Vitamin A supplements may not be helpful and may even cause toxicity. In this case, it's better to focus on consuming foods that are naturally rich in Vitamin A.

What am I missing if I'm not consuming enough Vitamin A?

Let us look at the important functions and health benefits of Vitamin A in detail in the next chapter.

2.

IMPORTANCE OF VITAMIN A

Vitamin A is involved in various physiological processes of the body. It plays various important roles through which it maintains the body's functions and prevents various diseases. First, let's see its important roles in the body.

Is Vitamin A an antioxidant?

Yes and no!

Yes, because Vitamin A enhances the antioxidant response of the body. And no, because Vitamin A is not directly involved in killing free radicals like true antioxidants. Instead, it regulates genes that help the body respond to and prevent oxidative stress. This is why Vitamin A can't technically be classified as a true antioxidant, it's more like an indirect antioxidant. While Vitamin A isn't technically a true antioxidant, it plays an important role in strengthening the body's antioxidant capacity and preventing the formation of harmful free radicals that can damage DNA. This can ultimately help prevent the onset of chronic diseases like diabetes, heart disease, cancer, respiratory issues, autoimmune disorders, infectious diseases, and neurological conditions.

Are carotenoids antioxidants?

Yes, carotenoids are true antioxidants. There are more than 500 different carotenoids, and most of them, including provitamin A carotenoids - beta-carotene, alpha-carotene, and beta-cryptoxanthin, are known for their antioxidant activity.

Carotenoids are very potent natural antioxidants. These carotenoids are highly effective at quenching singlet oxygen and scavenging reactive oxygen species found in cellular lipid bilayers. Beta-carotene, for instance, targets lipophilic radicals within each cell compartment and chelates oxygen-free radicals and eliminates their energy, thus avoiding peroxidation of lipids and guarding against damage caused by free radicals.

Due to their antioxidant properties, carotenoids can help reduce or even prevent the development of various free radical-related disorders, such as autoimmune diseases, cognitive disorders, diabetes, heart disease, and different types of cancer.

ROLE OF VITAMIN A IN THE BODY

The Important Anti-inflammatory Action of Vitamin A

Insufficient Vitamin A intake can cause inflammation and worsen existing inflammatory conditions. This deficiency may also contribute to the onset of Alzheimer's disease. In addition, persistent inflammation can lead to chronic ailments, including diabetes, heart disease, rheumatoid arthritis, cancer, and psoriasis.

Vitamin A is beneficial in various inflammatory issues, such as acne, Alzheimer's disease, bronchopulmonary dysplasia, and certain precancerous and cancerous states. This vitamin is regarded as an anti-inflammatory agent due to its vital role in strengthening the immune system. It helps regulate the immune system's response and prevent overreaction that may cause inflammation.

Vitamin A exists in three forms: retinol, retinal, and retinoic acid (RA), with the latter having the most biological activity. RA converts into two crucial derivatives, namely, 9-cis-retinoic acid and all-trans-retinoic acid (ATRA). Retinoid acids play a role in regulating the differentiation, maturation, and function of innate immune system cells, which is composed of macrophages and neutrophil. These cells respond immediately to pathogen invasion by activating natural killer T cells that carry out important immune regulatory functions. Macrophages include M1 macrophages that release pro-inflammatory cytokines and M2 macrophages that express anti-inflammatory factors. All-trans-retinoic acid (ATRA), a derivative of retinoid acid, can inhibit inflammatory responses by preventing macrophages from releasing inflammatory factors and inducing the conversion of M1 to M2 macrophages in the bone marrow.

Recent research has found that beta-carotene can help slow down the progression of rheumatoid arthritis. This is because beta-carotene inhibits the translocation of nuclear factor kappa B, reducing the transcription of pro-inflammatory cytokine genes such as interleukins and tumor necrosis factor-alpha (TNF-α). Beta-carotene is further converted into Vitamin A in the body, which is then metabolized into all-trans-retinoic acid (ATRA), which has anti-inflammatory properties. Consuming fruits and vegetables that are high in beta-carotene can have these positive effects, while supplements have been found to be ineffective.

What are the active forms of Vitamin A?

After you eat food, your body metabolizes Vitamin A and provitamin A into biologically active forms: retinol, retinal, and retinoic acid. Vitamin A exerts all of its action through these biologically active forms. All these three forms are toxic at high levels. Vitamin A levels can easily reach toxic levels when excessive Vitamin A supplements are taken. This is the reason why it is recommended to get Vitamin A from green and yellow vegetables, fruits, and dairy products rather than through dietary supplements.

Why is Vitamin A important?

Eyesight

Maintaining eye health is the most important and well-known function of Vitamin A. Having normal levels of Vitamin A is crucial for good vision, as having too much or too little can be harmful. Vitamin A plays a major role in the visual cycle and color vision, and its deficiency can cause vision loss and blindness.

Vitamin A is a component of the protein rhodopsin, a highly sensitive to the light pigment found in the retina within the eye. It allows the eyes to see in low-light environments, basically helping you see better in the dark. Vitamin A not only supports the vision function but also maintains the covering and lining of the eyes. It supports normal differentiation and function of the conjunctival membranes and cornea.

Another essential function of Vitamin A is that it is involved in visual phototransduction, which is the process that converts light into electrical signals. These signals from the retina travel through the optic nerve to the brain and are converted into an image.

Difficulty seeing in dim light is a characteristic of night blindness. It is an early sign of Vitamin A deficiency. If there are insufficient rhodopsin levels, the retina struggles to convert provitamin A carotenoids into Vitamin A, leading to temporary blindness in dark spots.

Inadequate intake of Vitamin A in the diet can gradually lead to complete vision loss over time. Vitamin A deficiency can cause dysfunction of the lining and covering of the eyes, leading to xerophthalmia or dry eyes. This condition can progress and even result in ulcers in the cornea, eventually causing blindness.

Skin Integrity

Vitamin A plays a vital role in maintaining the integrity and function of the skin. Vitamin A helps in the daily replacement of skin cells. Melanogenesis is the process by which melanocytes produce the pigment melanin, which provides skin color and protects deeper skin layers from the sun's DNA-damaging ultraviolet radiation. The phototransduction cascade, which initiates melanogenesis, requires Retinal (the active form of Vitamin A). In addition, retinoic acid regulates the melanocyte stem cells and influences melanocyte differentiation and proliferation. Vitamin A plays a crucial role in maintaining the integrity and function of the skin. Vitamin A helps in the daily replacement of skin cells. Melanogenesis is the process by which melanocytes produce the pigment melanin, which provides skin color and protects deeper skin layers from the sun's DNA-damaging ultraviolet radiation. The phototransduction cascade, which initiates melanogenesis, requires Retinal (the active form of Vitamin A). In addition, retinoic acid regulates the melanocyte stem cells and influences melanocyte differentiation and proliferation.

Hair Health

Vitamin A is an important micronutrient for hair growth. Vitamin A is essential for cell growth, which, in turn, helps your hair grow, but both too little and too much Vitamin A can have harmful effects. Retinoic acid, which is the biologically active form of Vitamin A, plays a significant role in regulating hair follicle stem cells and affecting the hair cycle's functioning. Additionally, Vitamin A aids in sebum production, which is a natural oil produced by skin glands on the scalp. Sebum helps hydrate the scalp, reduces frizz, and prevents breakage, ultimately promoting healthy hair growth.

Reproduction and Embryogenesis

Vitamin A metabolite, known as all-trans retinoic acid, plays a vital role in male and female reproductive systems, as well as in various events during the development of an embryo.

Moreover, Vitamin A is crucial for the upkeep of the male genital tract, aiding in the growth of sperm. Recent studies suggest that Vitamin A also supports the developing tissues of a fetus in the womb and aids in the formation of the placenta during pregnancy.

Cell Growth

Vitamin A is crucial in regulating the growth and differentiation of many types of cells. All cells are derived from stem cells and acquire their functions as they mature. Cell differentiation is the process by which cells acquire distinct roles as they divide. Vitamin A plays a role in cell proliferation, differentiation, and function by impacting the biosynthesis of various proteins, including those that regulate growth and cell function. Additionally, Vitamin A is involved in determining a cell's sensitivity to hormones and hormone-like factors. Studies suggest that Vitamin A also influences the production of secretory proteins that act as hormones.

Development Process (Central Nervous System)

Vitamin A is crucial for early development and signaling functions in the human brain and requires a delicate balance for optimal functioning. Retinoids, which are Vitamin A derivatives found in the central nervous system, regulate neuronal differentiation and neural tube patterning - the process by which cells in the developing nervous system gain specific identities.

Vitamin A plays a significant role in maintaining high function in the central nervous system and is essential for both the development and operation of the olfactory system. Retinoic acid, a Vitamin A metabolite, is involved in olfaction (sense of smell) and cognitive activities such as memory, learning, and spatial functions.

Studies have found lower levels of Vitamin A and beta-carotene in Alzheimer's disease (AD) patients. The degradation of retinoic acid signaling may influence the initiation and development of Alzheimer's disease. More importantly, research has shown that Vitamin A can slow the progression of Alzheimer's disease. Vitamin A has also been shown to protect against other brain diseases such as Parkinson's disease, cerebral ischemia, autism, and schizophrenia.

Bone Health

It was previously believed that Vitamin A increases bone resorption (breaking down of old bones) and prevents the building of new bones. If you take too much Vitamin A (more than 3,000 mcg or 10,000 IU/day), it can even increase the risk of fractures. However, recent studies have shown that not having enough Vitamin A can also increase the risk of fractures. More research has shown that Vitamin A (in the right amounts) can actually help promote healthy bones. Additionally, provitamin A (carotene and beta-cryptoxanthin) may also protect bones.

Carotene and beta-cryptoxanthin help with bone formation and can prevent the activation of nuclear factor-kappa B to inhibit the differentiation as well as maturation of osteoclasts (cells that break down bone). Both Vitamin A and provitamin A are important for building strong, healthy bones and can potentially prevent bone fractures.

Immunity

Vitamin A plays a vital role in immune system regulation. It protects against various infections and inflammatory and allergic diseases. Vitamin A deficiency increases your susceptibility to infection. All-trans-retinoic acid is the active form of Vitamin A, which has anti-inflammatory properties and is essential for generating both innate and adaptive immune cell responses. Vitamin A has an impact on the activation of neutrophils and macrophages. Additionally, it plays a significant role in regulating the differentiation of T-helper cells and B cells. In addition, Vitamin A has an important role in mucus secretion, providing the first line of defense against foreign bodies entering the body. Vitamin A provides mechanistic protection by playing an essential role in the formation and function of epithelial cells.

Red Blood Cell Formation

Retinoic acid, which is the active component of Vitamin A, regulates the hormone erythropoietin for a short period. Erythropoietin stimulates red blood cell production. Retinoids potentially control the programmed cell death of red blood cell precursors. Moreover, Vitamin A has the ability to enhance the mobility of iron from the liver to developing red blood cells, which helps in the incorporation of iron into hemoglobin. Hemoglobin is responsible for carrying oxygen in red blood cells.

Thyroid Function

Vitamin A reduces the risk of hypothyroidism. Vitamin A deficiency negatively impacts the thyroid health. Not enough Vitamin A in the body can cause the pituitary gland to create and release more thyroid-stimulating hormone (TSH). This can result in the thyroid gland becoming larger and less able to uptake iodine. Vitamin A activates thyroid hormone receptors, regulates thyroid hormone metabolism, and inhibits thyroid-stimulating hormone (TSH) secretion, thereby reducing the risk of goiter.

IN DISEASE PREVENTION AND TREATMENTS

As Vitamin A plays an important part in various physiological functions of the body, having enough Vitamin A can prevent and effectively be used in various disease treatments. Especially beta carotene from plant sources has more advanced protective effects than preformed Vitamin A. Let's see how Vitamin A is significant in different disease prevention and control:

Prevent Cancer

Vitamin A from plant sources is more effective in protecting against cancer than supplements. Some clinical trial suggests that Vitamin A supplements may reduce the risk of some cancers but at the same time increase the risk of other forms of cancer, such as prostate cancer, cardiovascular disease morbidity, and mortality. High-dose supplements of carotenoids may increase the risk of lung cancer in smokers.

Consuming a diet that is abundant in micronutrients, particularly Vitamin A, can boost the immune system and prognosis for individuals with head and neck cancer. It may also decrease the likelihood of developing oral and pharyngeal cancer.

Studies have suggested that Vitamin A and carotenoids have protective potential against the development of breast cancer. Vitamin A and carotenoids are potent antioxidants and are highly effective at scavenging free radicals, which helps to protect against photooxidative damage. They also protect breast cancer development and progression by inhibiting cell proliferation, survival, and invasion.

Acute Promyelocytic Leukemia

Myeloid stem cells in the bone marrow normally differentiate into platelets, red blood cells, and white blood cells (also known as leukocytes), which are crucial for the immune response. However, if myeloid cell differentiation is disrupted, it can lead to the overgrowth of immature white blood cells, causing leukemia. In people with Acute promyelocytic leukemia, administering high doses of all-trans retinoic acid (ATRA), an active metabolite of Vitamin A, can help restore normal differentiation and greatly improve chances of complete remission.

Measles

Measles is a viral infection that attacks the respiratory system and may spread to other parts of the body. It poses a serious threat to young children. One of the major risk factors for severe measles is a lack of Vitamin A. Consuming enough Vitamin A can help prevent measles and reduce mortality rates for those who contract the infection. World Health Organization recommends higher doses of Vitamin A to children over six months old who are malnourished, immunocompromised, or at risk of complications from measles.

Age-Related Macular Degeneration

Age-related macular degeneration (AMD) is an eye disease that can make your central vision blurry. The macula, which is responsible for sharp and direct vision and is a part of the retina (the tissue that is sensitive to light and located at the back of the eye), becomes damaged as you age. This condition is called age-related macular degeneration. As people get older, their risk of developing age-related macular degeneration increases, which is the most common cause of blindness in elderly people. This disease is complex and caused by genetic and environmental factors, such as aging, smoking, obesity, and high oxidative stress.

Vitamin A is an essential nutrient for the human eye and plays an important role in human retinal pigment epithelial cells. Several studies suggest a positive association between a reduction in dietary micronutrient intake and the progression of age-related macular degeneration. Micronutrients with antioxidant capacity may prevent oxidative stress involved in the development of degenerative eye diseases. The risk of macular degeneration can be effectively reduced by consuming foods rich in antioxidants such as beta-carotene, which has a protective effect on age-related macular degeneration. Long-term consumption of fruits and vegetables containing provitamin A carotenoid reduces the risk of any stage of AMD.

Prevention of Heart Disease

Cardiovascular disease (CVD) is a major cause of death worldwide, and its prevention is crucial. Vitamins, especially those with antioxidant properties, can play an essential role in preventing and treating cardiovascular disease. Vitamin A and provitamin A carotenoids can reduce oxidative stress by acting as antioxidants. The development of cardiovascular diseases is believed to be significantly influenced by oxidative stress.

Vitamin A and carotenoids possess anti-inflammatory and antioxidant properties, making them important for reducing the incidence of heart disease. These compounds are effective in mitigating and protecting against various forms of cardiovascular diseases, such as atherosclerosis, hypertension, arrhythmias, myocardial ischemia, and heart failure. Research indicates that high levels of Vitamin A in the body can reduce both systolic and diastolic blood pressure in individuals with hypertension.

Vitamin A can reduce atherosclerosis due to its antioxidant and anti-inflammatory properties. Reports indicate that Vitamin A can lower oxidative stress levels in diabetic patients with ischemic heart disease. Additionally, beta-carotene can reduce the size of ischemia-reperfusion-induced infarcts and improve post-ischemic cardiac function recovery.

Eating red, green, and orange vegetables and fruits can provide the heart-protective effects associated with Vitamin A. While taking vitamin supplements may not provide many cardiovascular benefits, getting Vitamin A and beta carotene from food is recommended.

Treating Skin Disorders

Vitamin A is used topically and taken orally to treat various skin conditions. From severe acne to premature aging, warts, and psoriasis, Vitamin A and its derivatives can work wonders for your skin.

In fact, Vitamin A was the first Vitamin Approved by the Food and Drug Administration as an anti-wrinkle agent. It can change the appearance of your skin surface and has anti-aging effects. Retinoids, which are derivatives of Vitamin A, play a crucial role in cell division, differentiation, and cell death. They can promote keratinocyte proliferation, which are skin cells that secrete keratin - a protein that protects against microbial invasion, shields against U.V. exposure, and maintains skin hydration.

Vitamin A strengthens the protective function of your skin, limits transepidermal water loss, and protects collagen against degradation. It's also been shown to have beneficial effects on skin diseases with disturbances of keratinization, such as psoriasis. In psoriasis, skin cells build up, forming scales and itchy and dry patches. Vitamin A can help improve psoriasis symptoms by reducing the formation of inflammation-causing proteins, cytokines, and interleukins.

Wound Healing

The growth and differentiation of various cell types within the skin are regulated by Vitamin A. It plays a crucial role in the inflammatory phase of wound healing. In damaged tissue, Vitamin A promotes the renewal of skin cells, accelerates the process of tissue regeneration, and helps in maintaining the structure of the epithelial layer. The process of epithelialization involves the migration of epithelial cells upwards to repair the wounded area. This process is vital to wound healing. Also, Vitamin A can reverse the inhibitory effects of anti-inflammatory steroids on wound healing. Vitamin A enhances the production of collagen type I and fibronectin, which are essential for tissue repair. It also increases the proliferation of keratinocytes, which are required to restore the epidermal barrier and fibroblasts, which are necessary for reducing the size of the wound.

Sunburn

Skin exposure to sunlight is crucial for the production of Vitamin D, but long-term exposure to UV-A radiation (315-400 nm) can penetrate deep layers of the skin epidermis and generate free radicals that lead to premature skin aging. Both Vitamin A and provitamin A carotenoids protect against the harmful effects of sunlight. Carotenoids, especially beta-carotene and canthaxanthin, act as protective agents for the skin by scavenging free radicals.

Your body stores Vitamin A in the form of retinyl esters, which are concentrated in the skin and can absorb ultraviolet radiation. Applying retinyl palmitate (a form of Vitamin A) topically is as effective as using a sunscreen with a sun protection factor 20 in preventing sunburn erythema and the formation of thymine dimers, which can cause DNA damage in the skin and ultimately lead to skin cancer.

3.

10 BEST FOODS RICH IN VITAMIN A

The shortcut rule to identify food rich in Vitamin A is RYG, i.e., Red, Yellow, and Green. Red, yellow, and green colored fruits and vegetables are good sources of vitamin A. Here are the top 10 foods that are high in Vitamin A.

1. Sweet Potato

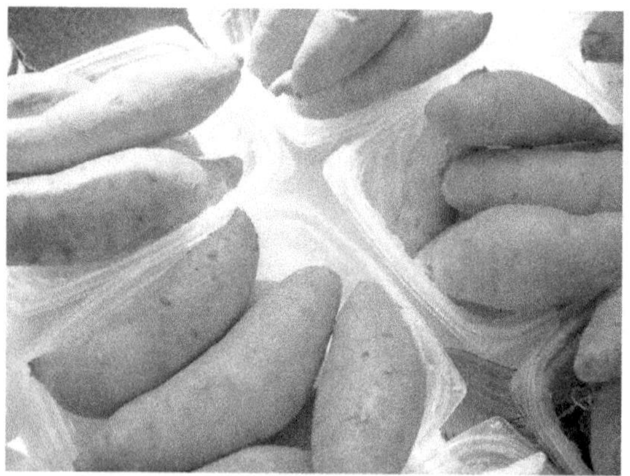

All varieties of sweet potatoes, orange, white, and purple, are good sources of vitamin A, but sweet potatoes with orange-yellow flesh are an excellent source of vitamin A because they have the highest levels of beta-carotene. One whole cooked orange sweet potato with the skin on provides 156% of the daily requirement for vitamin A. The deeper the orange color of the sweet potato, the more beta-carotene it contains. Beta carotene converts into vitamin A in the body and effectively reduces the risk of developing prostate cancer and colorectal cancer.

Purple fleshed sweet potatoes are low in beta-carotene and high in anthocyanin. This potent antioxidant may help reduce inflammation, improve neurological health, and protect against various non-communicable diseases.

Sweet potatoes are high in vitamin A as well as vitamin C, both of which are potent antioxidants that boost your immune system and protect against infection. The high fiber content of sweet potatoes promotes proper digestion and prevents constipation.

2. Spinach

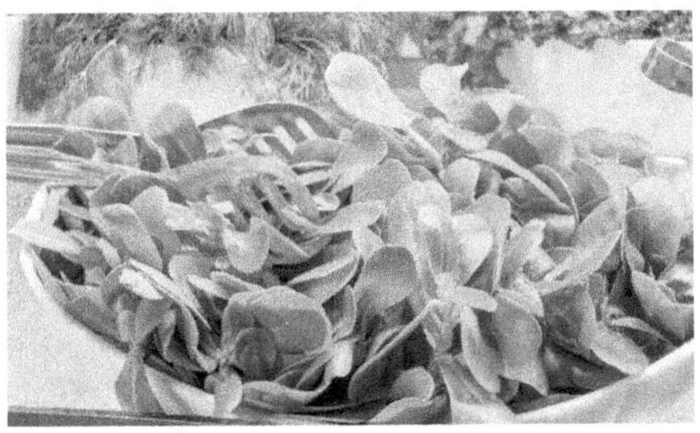

Spinach is a superfood because it is rich in many nutrients. Spinach is one of the best sources of Vitamin A. Half a cup of boiled spinach fulfills 64% of your daily vitamin A requirement. It not only improves vision and boosts your immune system but also prevents diabetes and high blood pressure. This leafy vegetable is also an excellent source of iron, calcium, and vitamin K. This means that by eating spinach regularly, you get strong bones and have thick hair and glowing skin. Spinach contains oxalates, which reduce the absorption of important nutrients of spinach in the body. To reduce the oxalate content of spinach, blanch it in enough water to reduce oxalate by 30%-87% and increase your body's absorption of nutrients.

3. Carrots

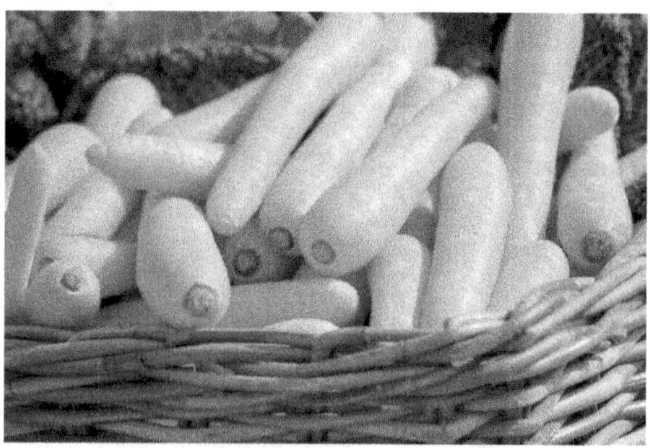

Carrots are rich in carotenoid antioxidants, especially beta-carotene. One cup or 100 grams of raw carrots fulfills 104% of your daily requirement of Vitamin A and keeps your eyes healthy. In addition to beta-carotene, carrots contain alpha-carotene that is partially metabolized into vitamin A in the body, as well as other potent antioxidants such as gamma-carotene, lutein (mostly in orange carrots), lycopene (mostly in red carrots), and zeaxanthin that reduce the risk of cancer and heart disease. Their soluble fiber content is high, which lowers cholesterol levels by binding to cholesterol particles and carrying them out of the body.

4. Pumpkin

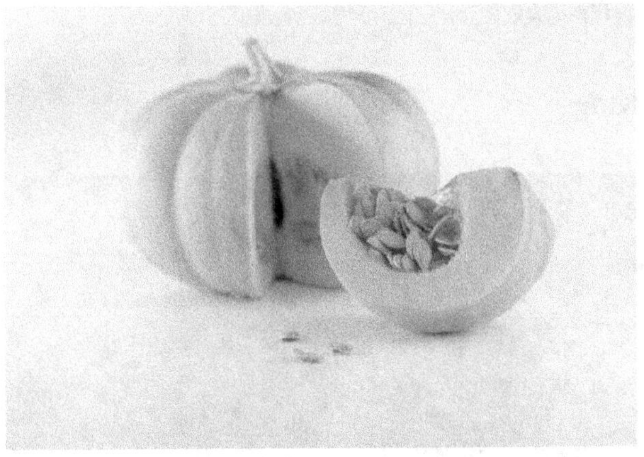

Pumpkin is an excellent source of beta-carotene. 100 grams of raw pumpkin fulfills 53% of your daily requirement of Vitamin A. Being high in beta-carotene, which eventually converts into vitamin A in the body, pumpkin lowers the risk of cataracts, strengthens your immune system, and provides protection against asthma. Along with vitamin A, pumpkin is also a good source of lutein and zeaxanthin. These two antioxidants fight free radicals in the body and reduce the risk of age-related macular degeneration. Pumpkin contains very few calories, which makes it weight-friendly. Instead of buying canned pumpkin purée, make the purée at home to avoid consuming excessive sugar and preservatives. You can make pumpkin pudding and pumpkin cake or use pumpkin purée as a pasta sauce.

Read 10 Smart Ways to Incorporate Pumpkin into Your Diet in the book Eat So What! Smart Ways to Stay Healthy.

5. Kale

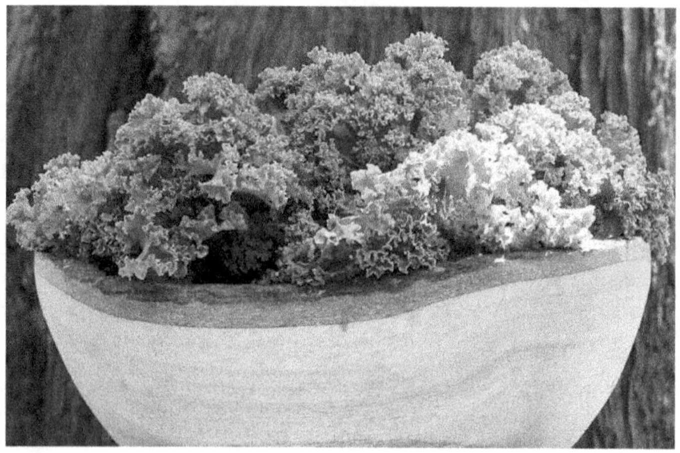

Kale is one of the healthiest vegetables. It is rich in many vitamins and minerals and is low in calories. 100 grams of raw kale contains 35% of the daily recommended value of vitamin A. Cooking reduces the vitamin A content of kale by up to 20%, so eat them raw to get the most vitamin A. Kale is also a good source of Vitamin C and K. Powerful antioxidants like quercetin and kaempferol present in kale help reduce the risk of cancer and heart disease.

If you have thyroid or kidney problems or are taking blood thinners, consult your doctor before including them in your diet. Consuming kale in excess hinders the functioning of the thyroid. Vitamin K plays a vital role in the process of blood clotting and interferes with blood-thinning medicines' activity. People with kidney problems should limit their intake of high-potassium vegetables like kale.

6. Muskmelon/ Cantaloupe Melon

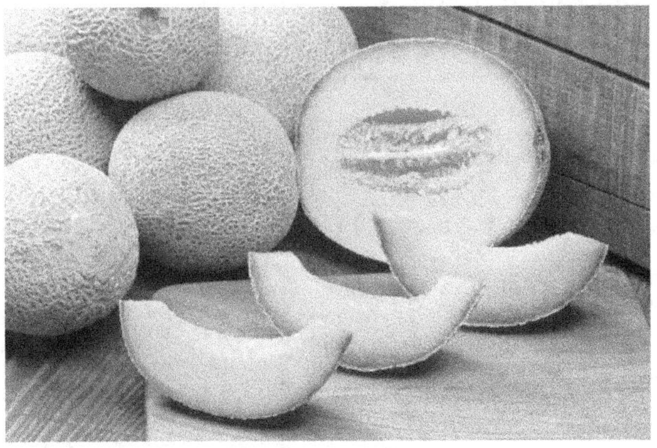

Cantaloupe is quite an underrated fruit. It is rich in beta carotene as well as vitamin C. 100 grams of raw cantaloupe provides 21% of the day's requirement of Vitamin A and 44% of Vitamin C. The best thing about cantaloupe is that it is mostly water and has zero fat and cholesterol. It also prevents and controls diabetes as well as high blood pressure. Watermelon is low in carbs and has a low glycemic index. It slowly releases glucose into the blood and does not allow blood sugar to rise, which makes it a diabetic-friendly fruit. Potassium-rich cantaloupe keeps your blood pressure under control and keeps your heart healthy. The high fiber and water content present in cantaloupe keeps your digestion healthy. Before cutting the melon, wash it thoroughly under running water and scrub the outer surface to remove any bacteria that may be present. Melons are known to be susceptible to contamination, so taking this precaution is important.

7. Red Bell Pepper

Red bell peppers is a great source of Vitamin A. Among green, yellow, and red bell peppers, bell peppers contain the most beta-carotene, which is converted into vitamin A in 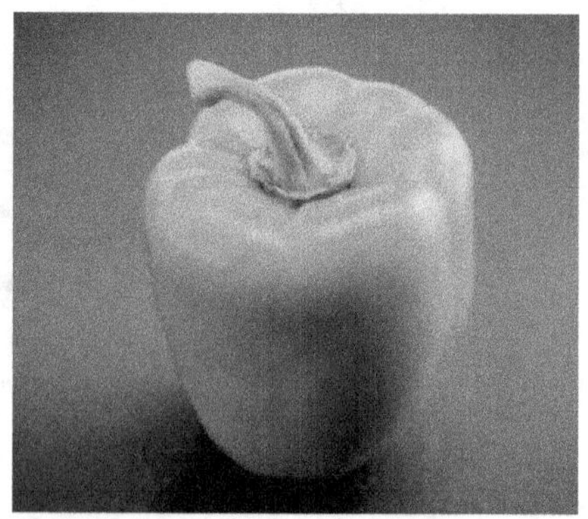 the body. 100 grams of red bell pepper fulfills 21% of the daily vitamin A requirement, almost 10 times more than green bell peppers. The red bell pepper is the fully ripened variety and the most nutritious of the three types. They are also a good vitamin C, potassium, magnesium, calcium, and iron source. Due to the high vitamin C content, red bell peppers help prevent anemia by increasing iron absorption in the body. However, the heat dilutes some of the health benefits of bell peppers, so eating it raw in a salad will give you maximum health benefits.

8. Cheese

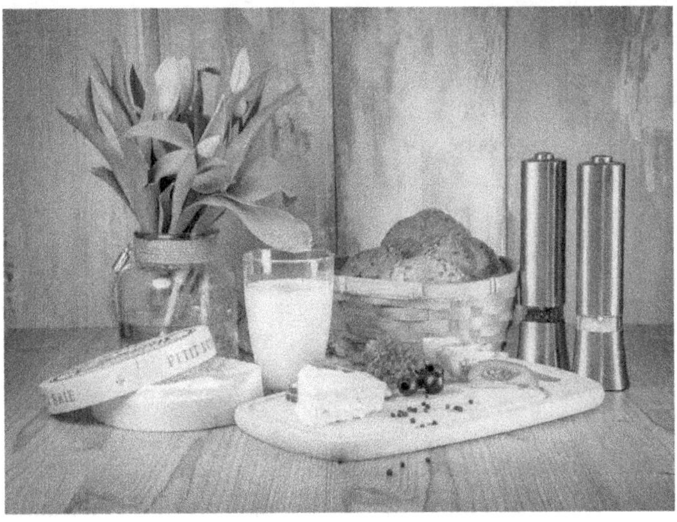

Although cheese isn't the healthiest source of vitamin A, at least you can eat cheese a little guilt-free. Unlike sugar, cheese isn't solely about calories, it also provides some nutrition. Ricotta cheese and cheddar cheese are good sources of vitamin A. 100 grams of Cheddar and

Ricotta cheese provide 45% and 18% of Vitamin A, respectively. This means 1 slice (17 grams) of cheddar and ricotta cheese provides 8% and 3% of vitamin A, respectively. Make sure you choose healthier varieties of cheese like cottage, ricotta, and cheddar instead of processed cheese. Avoid processed cheese completely as this variety has high calories and negligible health benefits, and it increases the cholesterol level in the body.

9. Mango

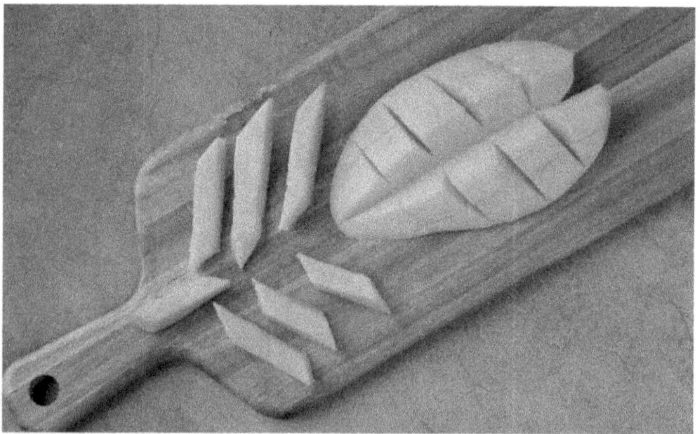

The summer season is incomplete without mangoes. They are not only delicious but also fulfill your daily requirement of Vitamin A. One whole mango contains 12% of the daily value of vitamin A. The high-water content and fiber in mangoes help in reducing constipation. A mango a day can stabilize your digestive system and help keep bowel movements normal. This sweet juicy fruit keeps your eyes healthy and boosts your immunity. Mango makes your bones strong and keeps your reproductive system healthy. Apart from vitamin A, mangoes are rich in vitamin C and folate.

10. Papaya

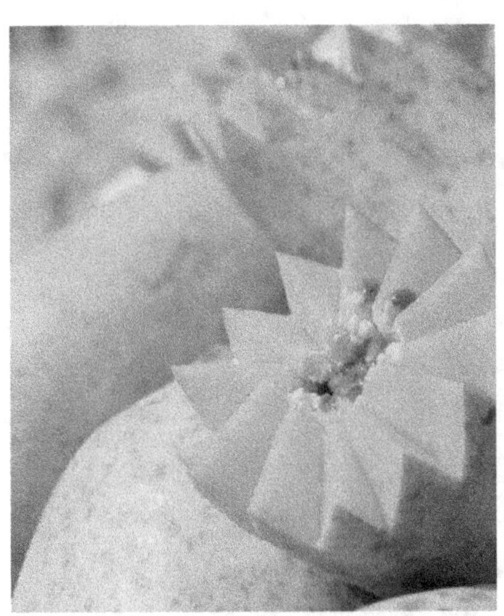

100 grams of papaya contains 9% of a day's recommended intake of vitamin A. Papaya is also an excellent Vitamin C source. 100 grams of papaya fulfills 75% of the Vitamin C requirement of the day. Papaya is low in calories, and about 88% of it consists of water, making it a favorable fruit for weight loss. Antioxidants like Vitamin A and C in papaya boost immunity, fight free radicals, and reduce inflammation in the body, thus preventing chronic diseases like heart disease and cancer. The high fiber content of papaya improves digestion by relieving constipation.

68

VITAMIN D

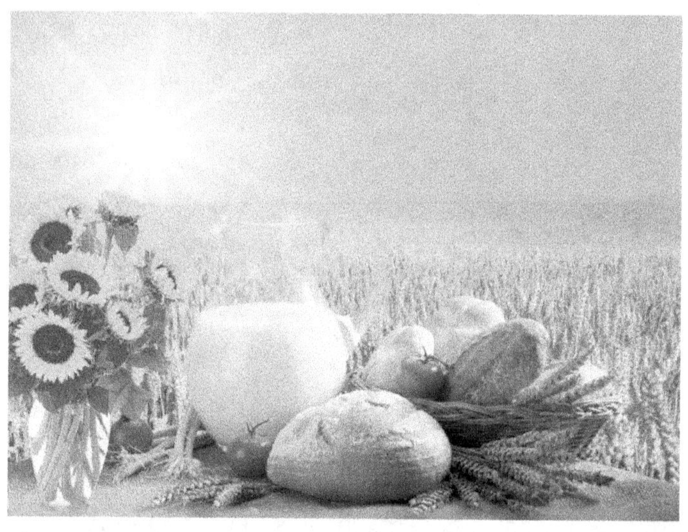

1.

EVERYTHING YOU NEED TO KNOW ABOUT VITAMIN D

Vitamin D is a fat-soluble essential vitamin, which is also known as calciferol. It is present in certain natural foods and can also be synthesized by the body when your skin is exposed to a certain range of ultraviolet rays from sunlight, which trigger vitamin D synthesis. Vitamin D cannot technically be considered an "essential" vitamin as it can be synthesized by the body. Non-essential doesn't mean it is not important, it simply means that your body can produce it, and you do not need to rely solely on food sources.

Read more about essential and non-essential nutrients in Eat So What! The Power of Vegetarianism.

Forms of Vitamin D

Vitamin D3 (cholecalciferol) and vitamin D2 (ergocalciferol) are the two most important forms of vitamin D for your health.

Vitamin D3 or Cholecalciferol (Animal-based) – It is naturally synthesized by animals, including humans. When your skin is exposed to ultraviolet rays from sunlight, it synthesizes cholecalciferol in the lower layers of the epidermis (skin) through a chemical reaction. Vitamin D3 is slightly more active than Vitamin D2.

Vitamin D2 or Ergocalciferol (Plant-based) – It can be found in food and is also used as a dietary supplement. Just like humans, some foods, such as mushrooms, make Vitamin D when exposed to ultraviolet light. The difference is our skin makes Vitamin D3, while mushrooms produce Vitamin D2 when exposed to ultraviolet rays of sunlight.

Vitamin D obtained from sun exposure and foods, i.e., both Vitamin D2 and D3 are biologically inactive and must get activated in the body. The first activation occurs in the liver, which converts vitamin D to 25-hydroxyvitamin D or 25(OH)D or, simply known as calcifediol. The second activation occurs primarily in the kidney and forms the physiologically active 1,25-dihydroxyvitamin D or 1,25(OH)2D or, simply known as calcitriol.

Which is more important for me, Vitamin D2 or D3?

Vitamin D3 and D2 both are important to health. So, you need both forms equally. However, it has been found that Vitamin D3 (cholecalciferol) is slightly more effective than Vitamin D2 (ergocalciferol) in increasing blood concentrations of the vitamin, and with the same daily doses of vitamin D2 and D3, calcifediol blood levels increased by vitamin D2 declined faster than the vitamin D3. So, it is basically Vitamin D3 that maintains the required levels of Vitamin D in your body. That makes getting sunlight even more crucial than obtaining Vitamin D from other sources. However, this does not diminish the importance of Vitamin D2. Both forms are equally important, but obtaining Vitamin D through sunlight can maintain your vitamin D levels for a longer period, and you get the maximum health benefits of vitamin D.

How much vitamin D do I need in a day?

The average daily recommended intake of vitamin D that is sufficient to meet the nutrient needs of nearly all (97%–98%) healthy individuals is:

Age 0-12 months – 400 IU (10 mcg) [Adequate Intake (AI)]

Age 1 - 70 years – 600 IU (15 mcg)

Age 70+ years – 800 IU (20 mcg)

*1 mcg is equal to 40 IU

How common is Vitamin D deficiency?

It would seem that Vitamin D is probably the easiest nutrient to get because it doesn't even need to depend on food, and you can easily get it from the sunlight, but in reality, about 50% of the world's population is vitamin D deficient. One of the most prevalent reasons for this is that many individuals do not receive adequate sunlight. This could be due to spending more time indoors and applying sunscreen before going outdoors.

What are the reasons that lead to a deficiency in Vitamin D?

- You are not getting enough sunlight exposure.

- Your diet might be lacking in vitamin D.

- You might have a malabsorption problem, which makes your body unable to absorb enough vitamin D from food.

- You live in a colder area.

- Your liver or kidneys are unable to convert vitamin D to its active form as all vitamin D forms are inactive in general and get activated in the liver and kidney.

- You have had weight loss surgery.

- You might be taking other medications that are interfering with how your body converts or absorbs vitamin D.

- You have certain medical conditions, such as liver disease or kidney disease.

What are the risk factors associated with vitamin D deficiency?

Fat Malabsorption: Fat malabsorption is a condition where your body is unable to absorb certain nutrients from your diet, even if you eat nutrient-dense foods. This can be caused by various factors such as lactose intolerance, prolonged use of antibiotics, damage to the intestine due to infection, inflammation or surgery, certain medical conditions, and radiation therapy. Vitamin D is a fat-soluble nutrient, which means that its absorption depends on the intestine's ability to absorb dietary fat. If you have difficulty absorbing dietary fat, your vitamin D levels might be low, and you may need to take vitamin D supplements.

Obesity: Studies have found that people who have a body mass index (BMI) of 30 or higher tend to have lower vitamin D levels than lean people. While obesity does not hinder your skin's ability to produce vitamin D, having more subcutaneous fat can absorb more of the vitamin, making it less available in the body. Therefore, People who are obese need to consume more vitamin D in order to achieve similar levels to those with a normal weight.

Gastric Bypass Surgery: Individuals who are obese and have had a gastric bypass surgery may become vitamin D deficient. It is because, during this procedure, a portion of the upper small intestine responsible for absorbing vitamin D is bypassed. As a result, vitamin D that is released from fat stores into the bloodstream may not elevate the levels of 25(OH)D (the active form of vitamin D) to a sufficient level over time.

Kidney or Liver Disease: Kidney or liver disease can affect your body's ability to convert inactive vitamin D into active forms for use.

Certain Medical Conditions: Some medical conditions like certain liver diseases, celiac disease, Crohn's disease, cystic fibrosis, and ulcerative colitis can lead to fat malabsorption. This affects the gut's ability to absorb vitamin D from food. Individuals with these conditions have a higher risk of vitamin D deficiency. Because of these conditions, they may also avoid certain foods like dairy products or consume them in small amounts, which can contribute to vitamin D deficiency.

Certain Medications: Using stimulant laxatives for an extended period can decrease the body's ability to absorb vitamin D from food, and taking high doses can even lead to osteomalacia.

Individuals who take oral antidiabetic medication typically have lower levels of vitamin D compared to those with diabetes who do not take these drugs.

Other medications that affect vitamin D status are steroids, weight-loss drugs, anti-seizure drugs, antivirals, antidepressants, anti-hypertensive drugs, vitamin K antagonists, and bile acid sequestrants.

What health problems can occur from Vitamin D deficiency?

Low blood levels of vitamin D are associated with the following conditions:

Hypocalcemia

Low levels of calcium in your blood can result in a condition known as hypocalcemia. Having sufficient levels of calcium is essential for maintaining strong and healthy bones, as well as a healthy functioning heart. When the body lacks vitamin D, your body cannot absorb enough calcium to meet its requirements. Therefore, a deficiency in vitamin D can cause low calcium levels in the blood, which can result in weakened bones and impact cardiovascular health.

Hypophosphatemia

If your body has low levels of phosphate, you may have a short-term or chronic condition called hypophosphatemia. Phosphate is vital for building and repairing bones and teeth, enabling muscle contraction, and ensuring nerve function. While vitamin D status doesn't directly impact phosphate levels, it can indirectly affect them. A lack of vitamin D in the body reduces calcium absorption, causing hypocalcemia. This, in turn, stimulates the secretion of parathyroid hormone (PTH) to fix the hypocalcemia by acting on bone and kidney. However, it also increases urinary phosphate excretion, leading to hypophosphatemia and osteomalacia.

Rickets

Rickets is a medical condition that primarily affects children and results in softening and weakening of the bones. This is usually due to a severe and prolonged deficiency of vitamin D.

Vitamin D is necessary for maintaining bone health. Adequate calcium and phosphate availability in the body is necessary for normal bone development and mineralization. Vitamin D plays an important role in promoting the absorption of calcium and phosphorus, which is necessary for bone mineralization. When calcium and phosphate levels are insufficient, vitamin D stimulates bone resorption to maintain serum calcium and phosphorus levels. However, in the case of vitamin D deficiency, there is not enough vitamin D available in the body to maintain optimum calcium and phosphorus levels, resulting in hypocalcemia and hypophosphatemia.

This deficient mineralization can lead to rickets and/or osteomalacia. Rickets occur when there is deficient mineralization in the growth plate, whereas osteomalacia is characterized by deficient mineralization of the bone matrix. These conditions cause the bones to become weak and bend over time.

Osteomalacia

Osteomalacia is a condition in adults where bones soften due to a prolonged deficiency of vitamin D. This results in impaired mineralization of bone matrix, which leads to weakened bones that are more susceptible to fractures.

Osteoporosis

Osteoporosis is a condition where the density and mass of bones decrease, or the quality and structure of bones change. This can cause bones to become weak and increase the likelihood of fractures.

Studies have found that insufficient intake of vitamin D over a prolonged period can cause demineralization of bones. A lack of vitamin D results in reduced absorption of calcium. The parathyroid glands respond by producing excess parathyroid hormone (PTH), leading to hyperparathyroidism. This eventually causes the body to extract calcium from bones to maintain calcium levels in the bloodstream. Continuous bone resorption weakens bone architecture, increasing the risk of fractures and ultimately resulting in osteoporosis and elevated fracture risk.

Cardiovascular Disease

Having low levels of vitamin D can increase your chances of developing cardiovascular diseases such as hypertension, heart failure, and ischemic heart disease. Vitamin D is important in regulating blood pressure as it hinders the secretion of renin and the activation of RAAS, which leads to a reduction in the level of angiotensin II, the main culprit in raising blood pressure. In people with vitamin D deficiency, the level of angiotensin II increases, leading to hypertension. Furthermore, heart patients suffering from severe vitamin D deficiency are at a higher risk of sudden cardiac death or heart failure compared to those with optimal levels of vitamin D.

Lower levels of vitamin D are also linked to a higher risk of diabetes. A study was conducted on individuals with impaired fasting glucose to determine the impact of vitamin D on fasting glucose levels. The study concluded that individuals with normal levels of vitamin D experienced a lesser increase in fasting glucose levels compared to those with low levels of vitamin D. This indicates that vitamin D might play a crucial role in regulating glycemic control, leading to potential benefits for cardiovascular outcomes.

Severe Asthma

Vitamin D not only can prevent asthma, but it also prevents the worsening of asthma. Low levels of Vitamin D may increase the frequency of asthma attacks and wheezing and require more medication. This is because low levels of Vitamin D can increase airway smooth muscle (ASM), causing narrowing of the airway and reducing lung function in severe asthma. To prevent and control asthma, it's important to get your daily dose of Vitamin D from natural sources like sun exposure and food. However, taking Vitamin D supplements may not produce the same results and can even worsen asthma symptoms.

Cognitive Impairment

Low Vitamin D levels can lead to a higher chance of cognitive decline. Vitamin D is a hormone that is important for the central nervous system. It helps regulate neurotransmitters and neurotrophins and has protective properties for the brain. Vitamin D also helps increase nerve growth factor levels and clears out amyloid. Studies have shown that people with cognitive impairment and dementia have lower levels of Vitamin D. It is because, when there is a deficiency of Vitamin D in the body, nerve growth factor levels decrease and amyloid accumulates, which can increase the risk of developing cognitive impairment, dementia, and Alzheimer's disease.

Cancer

Research has linked low levels of Vitamin D to various types of cancer, such as prostate, breast cancer, colon cancer, and multiple myeloma. This is because Vitamin D is known to have various biological functions that may help prevent or reduce the progression of cancer. These functions include inhibiting cancer cell growth, slowing down tumor progression, and inducing cancer cell death (apoptosis).

Autoimmune Disorders

A deficiency in Vitamin D can increase your risk of autoimmune diseases such as rheumatoid arthritis, type 1 diabetes, systemic lupus erythematosus, multiple sclerosis, and inflammatory bowel disease.

Vitamin D has the ability to regulate gene expression and inflammation, which can have a positive impact on the immune system. It has been proven to reduce the production of pro-inflammatory cytokines, enhance Treg activity, improve Natural Killer T cell function, and promote the production of anti-inflammatory cytokines. Insufficient Vitamin D intake can contribute to the development and progression of autoimmune disorders.

Infections

Research has shown that a deficiency in Vitamin D increases the risk and severity of respiratory infections such as colds, tuberculosis, pneumonia, and bronchitis. Vitamin D plays a vital role in regulating the immune system, it modulates both innate and adaptive immune responses. It also influences the production of an important antimicrobial peptide, cathelicidin.

Vitamin D helps to decrease the production of inflammation-causing cytokines while increasing the production of anti-inflammatory and anti-allergic cytokines. Furthermore, it increases the production of cathelicidin, which is an antimicrobial peptide that can directly eliminate pathogens. In addition to its role against Mycobacterium tuberculosis, cathelicidin has also been found to be effective against viruses and other bacteria.

If you are deficient in Vitamin D, your immune system becomes dysregulated and more prone to a pro-inflammatory state, which increases your susceptibility to infections caused by bacteria and viruses.

Pregnancy Complications

Maintaining normal Vitamin D levels during pregnancy is crucial for both mother's and child's health. Vitamin D aids in calcium absorption in your body, which is important for both children and adults. In the third trimester of pregnancy, there is an increase in calcium demands, making vitamin D status vital for optimal maternal health, fetal bone growth, and positive outcomes for both mother and child. If there is a deficiency of vitamin D during pregnancy, it can lead to various complications such as preeclampsia (hypertension during pregnancy), low birth weight, hypocalcemia and poor growth in the baby, weak bones, and an increased risk of autoimmune diseases.

How do I know if I am deficient in vitamin D?

It is possible to have a vitamin D deficiency without experiencing any symptoms. Here are some common symptoms associated with vitamin D deficiency:

- Fatigue and exhaustion
- Muscle cramps and muscle weakness
- Bone pain
- Mood changes, sadness, or depression
- Improper sleeping pattern
- Hair loss
- Loss of appetite

What should I do if I have symptoms of Vitamin D deficiency?

If you are experiencing exhaustion, pain in bones and muscles, or other vitamin D deficiency symptoms, consult your doctor. Your doctor might request a calcifediol blood test to check if there are any deficiencies of Vitamin D in your bloodstream.

What is a calcifediol blood test?

The blood concentration of calcifediol or 25(OH)D3 is considered the best indicator of vitamin D status, this is why the calcifediol blood test is used to determine how much actual vitamin D is in your body.

Calcifediol is measured in nanograms per milliliter (ng/mL). Different countries follow different guidelines for vitamin D intake. Some professional societies recommend a standard range of between 20 ng/mL and 40 ng/mL, while others recommend a normal range of between 30 and 50 ng/mL.

2.

IMPORTANCE OF VITAMIN D

FUNCTIONS OF VITAMIN D IN THE BODY

Role in Absorption of Calcium and Phosphorous

Vitamin D is crucial for strong bones. Calcium and phosphorous are essential minerals that help make bones strong. Vitamin D plays an essential role in absorbing and balancing calcium and phosphorous in the body, which enhances bone mineralization and increases bone mineral density (BMD).

Bone mineralization is the process of filling organic bones with calcium and phosphate. The higher the density of calcium and phosphate in your bones, the more robust and less prone to breaking they become.

Vitamin D primarily enhances the absorption of calcium and phosphorus in the small intestine. When calcium levels are low, Parathyroid Hormone (PTH) secretion increases, which stimulates the production of vitamin D active metabolite in the kidney. This hormone interacts with the vitamin D receptor [VDR] in the intestine, increasing calcium absorption. As a result, serum calcium and phosphorus concentrations increase, which are necessary for the mineralization of bones to prevent rickets, osteomalacia, and osteoporosis.

If normal blood calcium levels are not maintained through intestinal calcium absorption, vitamin D metabolite works with PTH to increase calcium reabsorption from the kidney and may remove calcium from the bones to maintain optimal physiological levels.

Vitamin D deficiency leads to a decrease in calcium absorption and release of calcium from the bones to maintain circulating calcium concentrations. This causes bones to weaken and become more susceptible to breaking.

Is Vitamin D an Antioxidant?

While current research studies have not confirmed vitamin D's potential role as an antioxidant, several studies have found that it effectively regulates oxidative stress. Both Vitamin D3 and Vitamin D2 can inhibit iron-dependent liposomal lipid peroxidation. Vitamin D helps to reduce oxidative stress by promoting the production of various molecules that play a role in the body's antioxidant defense system. It enhances the expression of the body's master antioxidant, Glutathione, and other antioxidant enzymes, including glutathione peroxidase and superoxide dismutase enzymes. Additionally, it suppresses the expression of free radical-producing NADPH oxidase, which helps prevent chronic diseases like diabetes, cardiovascular disease, and chronic kidney disease.

Anti-inflammatory Action

The role of Vitamin D in regulating the inflammation system is crucial. It helps control the production of inflammatory cytokines, prostaglandins, immune cells, and the nuclear factor kappa B (NF-κB) pathway, which are vital in developing immune-related diseases.

Vitamin D has powerful anti-inflammatory properties and can reduce pro-inflammatory mediators and increase anti-inflammatory cytokines. It regulates the adaptive immune system, particularly T cells, which can differentiate into pro-inflammatory TH1 cytokine cells or anti-inflammatory TH2 cytokine cells. Vitamin D suppresses inflammation causing TH1 proliferation and cytokine production while also increasing anti-inflammatory TH2 cell proliferation and cytokine production.

In addition, Vitamin D plays a crucial role in the Nuclear factor kappa B pathway (NF-κB), a major regulator of immune, stress, and inflammatory responses. The NFκB pathway can upregulate the expression of pro-inflammatory cytokines and contribute to the induction of C-reactive protein (CRP), a marker of inflammation in the body. Vitamin D can exert an anti-inflammatory effect by modulating the NFκB pathway and decreasing CRP levels. It can inhibit NF-κB activation by upregulating IκBα, the inhibitor of NF-κB, which decreases pro-inflammatory cytokine levels. Vitamin D can also inhibit the synthesis of inflammation-causing Prostaglandin E2 (PGE2).

Neuroprotective Action

Research has shown that Vitamin D plays a vital role in protecting the nervous system from injury and neurotoxicity. A deficiency in Vitamin D may increase the risk of various central nervous system (CNS) diseases such as dementia, schizophrenia, and multiple sclerosis.

Vitamin D. regulates the development and function of the nervous system It has a neuroprotective effect by influencing the production and release of growth factors neurotrophin, synthesis of neuro mediators that transmit messages between neurons, neuronal calcium regulation, an essential role in glutamatergic systems, and prevention of oxidative damage to nerve cells.

Oxidative stress is the leading cause of various neurodegenerative diseases, and Vitamin D3 has been found to alleviate oxidative stress and provide neuroprotection. It decreases lipid peroxidation, improves the GST enzyme activity, and increases the amount of reduced Glutathione, thereby reducing the effects of oxidative stress.

Immunomodulatory Effects of Vitamin D

Vitamin D has the ability to change how your immune system responds, making it an immunomodulator. Normally, the immune system fights off pathogens and foreign substances. However, sometimes, it can overreact due to a false alarm, causing an imbalance in the body and leading to autoimmune diseases. Immunomodulators help prevent this by regulating the immune system's response to achieve an immune balance.

Vitamin D's immunomodulatory effect is based on its ability to modify gene transcription. It can downregulate all adaptive immunity mechanisms, reduce inflammation, and increase immunological tolerance. Vitamin D also restricts T cell overreaction to an antigen, which impairs B cell activity and antibody production. Moreover, it influences cytokine production by reducing inflammation-causing cytokine production and stimulating immune cells to release more anti-inflammatory cytokines.

Top health benefits of getting Vitamin D from natural sources:

Prevent Osteoporosis

Osteoporosis is a frequently occurring bone disease among individuals who are 65 years or older. This condition arises from changes in bone mineral density and mass, which lead to a decline in bone structure and quality. This, in turn, reduces bone strength, putting individuals at a higher risk of experiencing fractures.

Osteoporosis stems from inflammation and muscle dysfunction. Elevated levels of inflammation-causing cytokines in the body are linked to increased bone metabolism. Vitamin D helps reduce the risk of bone fractures through various mechanisms, it enhances muscle strength, which helps decrease the frequency of falls, a major contributor to fractures. Additionally, vitamin D's anti-inflammatory and immunoregulatory actions help lower the production of cytokines that cause inflammation. This, in turn, reduces bone turnover and increases bone mineral density, thereby strengthening bones and minimizing fracture risk.

Prevent Hypertension

Vitamin D plays a vital role in regulating the renin-angiotensin-aldosterone system, thereby decreasing blood pressure by reducing the blood pressure-raising hormone, angiotensin II. Another hormone, Parathyroid hormone (PTH), increases systolic blood pressure by decreasing systemic vascular resistance, increasing heart rate, and elevating cardiac output. Vitamin D lowers PTH concentrations and leads to decreased systolic and diastolic blood pressure. However, clinical trials indicate that taking vitamin D supplements may not reduce cardiovascular risks.

Prevent Cardiovascular Diseases

Your vitamin D status is closely connected to your heart health and the likelihood of developing cardiovascular disease. A deficiency in vitamin D can lead to arterial stiffening, high cholesterol levels, vascular dysfunction, and an increased risk of strokes. Those with low levels of vitamin D are twice as likely to have a heart attack as those with high levels. Vitamin D helps regulate immune cells and inflammatory pathways that contribute to cardiovascular disease conditions such as atherosclerosis. Additionally, vitamin D plays a vital role in regulating cholesterol levels, one of the primary risk factors for cardiovascular disease.

Vitamin D's influence on calcium metabolism is crucial, as it promotes intestinal calcium absorption, reduces intestinal fatty acid absorption, and facilitates the conversion of cholesterol into bile acids in the liver, leading to lower cholesterol levels. Vitamin D also impacts lipoprotein metabolism, lowering triglyceride synthesis and secretion in the liver and leading to reduced triglyceride and VLDL-C levels and increased HDL-C levels (good cholesterol).

Lower Risk of Diabetes

Low levels of vitamin D have been linked to higher levels of inflammation in the body, which in turn could lead to insulin resistance and type 2 diabetes. Fortunately, getting enough vitamin D from natural sources can help prevent type 2 diabetes or improve insulin release and insulin sensitivity. However, clinical studies have shown that taking vitamin D supplements doesn't have a significant impact on blood sugar control. So, the diabetes-preventive benefits of vitamin D are best achieved by obtaining vitamin D from sunlight and a diet rich in vitamin D rather than from dietary supplements.

Prevent Cancer

Consuming high amounts of Vitamin D can significantly reduce the risk of cancer types, such as breast, prostate, and colon cancer, and lower cancer mortality rates.

Vitamin D has several biological functions that can help prevent or slow down cancer development. These include reducing cancer cell growth, decreasing tumor progression, and limiting tumor blood vessel formation (angiogenesis). Additionally, Vitamin D has anti-inflammatory and immunomodulatory effects.

When it comes to cancer-related inflammation, Vitamin D can help by decreasing levels of cyclooxygenase-2 (COX-2) enzyme, which is responsible for the production of inflammatory prostaglandins. Vitamin D also boosts the enzyme that breaks down prostaglandins, leading to decreased levels of these inflammatory mediators. Vitamin D also suppresses the activation and signaling of a protein called NFκB, which promotes inflammation and contributes to the development of cancer.

Moreover, Vitamin D can also help the immune system fight cancer by suppressing the function of Myeloid-derived suppressor cells (MDSC), which inhibit the ability of T cells to attack and remove tumor cells from the body. By reducing MDSC activity, Vitamin D can increase T-cell mediated clearance of cancer cells.

Prevent Rheumatoid Arthritis

The immune system's primary function is to protect the body from infections. However, in cases of autoimmune conditions such as rheumatoid arthritis, the immune system erroneously attacks the healthy cells in the joints, lungs, and other areas. Studies have shown that individuals with higher levels of vitamin D have a lower risk of developing autoimmune diseases. This is attributed to vitamin D's ability to interact with immune cells, alter the response of the immune system, and regulate inflammation-regulating genes. Consequently, the body is better equipped to fight off sickness and disease, including arthritis.

Improve Eczema (Atopic Dermatitis)

Skin inflammation and immune dysfunction can lead to damage to the skin barrier and increase the likelihood of skin infections and atopic dermatitis (eczema). Vitamin D is known to have a regulatory effect on both immune function and the skin barrier.

Individuals with eczema often lack the proper production of effector cells of innate immunity, including antimicrobial peptides like cathelicidin. Vitamin D can enhance the production of cathelicidin, which boosts antimicrobial activity. Additionally, vitamin D can directly suppress skin inflammation by increasing the levels of the anti-inflammatory cytokine IL-10.

Regarding skin barrier function, vitamin D plays a regulatory role in controlling cell growth in the deepest skin layer, regulating proteins in this layer, and synthesizing lipids necessary for the skin's barrier function. Therefore, vitamin D has the potential to improve allergy outcomes through its effects on epidermal barrier function, immune regulation, and bacterial defense.

Promote Weight Loss

Although there is no clear evidence that consuming higher amounts of vitamin D directly leads to weight loss, it can still help support your weight loss journey if combined with exercise and a nutritious diet. Vitamin D can affect the way fat is formed and stored in your body and increase levels of serotonin and testosterone. Serotonin is known to impact mood, emotional stability, and sleep and acts as a hunger suppressant, increasing satiety and controlling appetite. Meanwhile, testosterone plays a vital role in boosting metabolism, burning more calories, and aiding in weight loss.

Prevent Depression and Enhance Mood

Research has shown that low vitamin D levels may be linked to anxiety and depression. This is because vitamin D is crucial in serotonin production, a neurotransmitter that elevates your mood, emotions, happiness, and sexual behavior.

Improve Sleep Quality

A deficiency in Vitamin D can increase your likelihood of experiencing sleep disorders. This is because Vitamin D is crucial in regulating sleep and improving the production of melatonin, which is known as the sleep hormone. Melatonin levels naturally increase in the evening, helping to calm the body and promote sleep. Ensuring that your diet includes sufficient Vitamin D-rich foods and exposure to sunlight can have a positive impact on preventing, managing, or even correcting sleep disorders. This can result in a decrease in the time it takes to fall asleep, better overall sleep quality, and longer sleep duration.

3.

10 NATURAL SOURCES TO GET VITAMIN D

Spending time in the early morning sunlight is the best way to your daily dose of Vitamin D. While it can be tough to get enough vitamin D from your diet alone, it's also important to eat foods high in this nutrient to avoid any deficiencies. Getting enough vitamin D is important for your health, and although sunlight exposure is the best way to achieve this, it may not always be possible to get enough during the winter months. That's why it's essential to include foods high in vitamin D in your diet. While not all foods listed below can provide enough vitamin D when taken alone, combining them can help you meet your daily requirements. Moreover, these foods offer other nutrients and fiber that can boost your overall health. Unlike supplements, there is no risk of vitamin D toxicity from either sunlight exposure or consuming foods rich in vitamin D. So, even if you're currently taking supplements for a vitamin D deficiency, it's better to switch to natural sources once your course is complete.

Below are the 10 natural sources to get vitamin D:

1. Sunlight

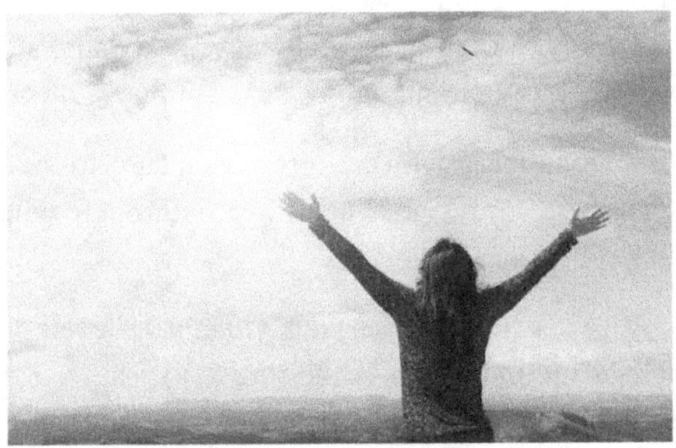

Many individuals aren't getting enough sunlight, perhaps due to spending more time indoors or using sunscreen when outside. However, it's important to note that sunlight is unbeatable when it comes to obtaining sufficient amounts of vitamin D. To safely receive this vitamin from the sun without risking sunburn or harmful UV radiation, follow these steps:

• It's important to get 10-25 minutes of sunlight exposure before noon, as the ultraviolet B rays with a wavelength of 290-320 nanometers during this time period are necessary for the skin to create vitamin D.

• When the skin is exposed to sunlight, it triggers the production of vitamin D within the body.

• The longer you're exposed to the sun, the more vitamin D your body produces. However, be careful not to overdo it, as excessive sunlight can lead to sunburn and other skin issues.

• It is important to have daily exposure to the sun in order to receive enough vitamin D. However if this is not possible, it is recommended to have sun exposure at least twice a week for a minimum of 25-30 minutes.

• It is recommended to get direct exposure to sunlight rather than the rays that are filtered through window glasses.

• If you want to increase your vitamin D levels while spending time in the sun, make sure to expose your face, arms, and hands or an equivalent area of your body.

• During this period, it is recommended that you avoid using sunscreen because it blocks the sun rays from entering your skin. However, remember to wear sunscreen whenever you leave home.

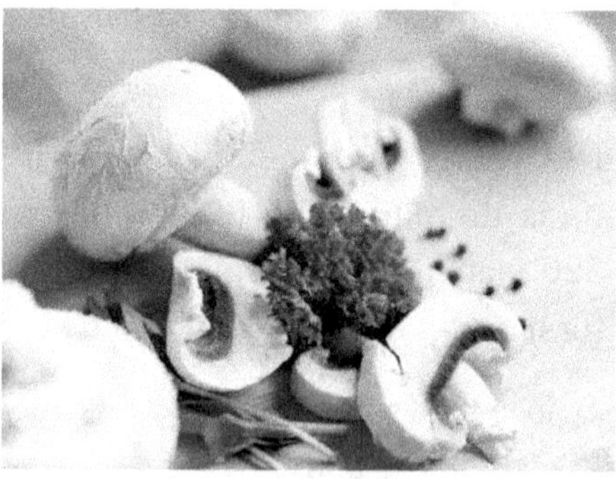

2. Mushrooms

Like humans, mushrooms can synthesize vitamin D when exposed to sunlight. When exposed to UV light, the ergosterol in mushrooms is converted to vitamin D. Next time you plan to eat mushrooms, expose them to sunlight for about 10-15 minutes in the morning to make them rich in Vitamin D. You can eat fried mushrooms and can also use them as a filling for sandwiches or add to noodles.

3. Whole Cow's Milk

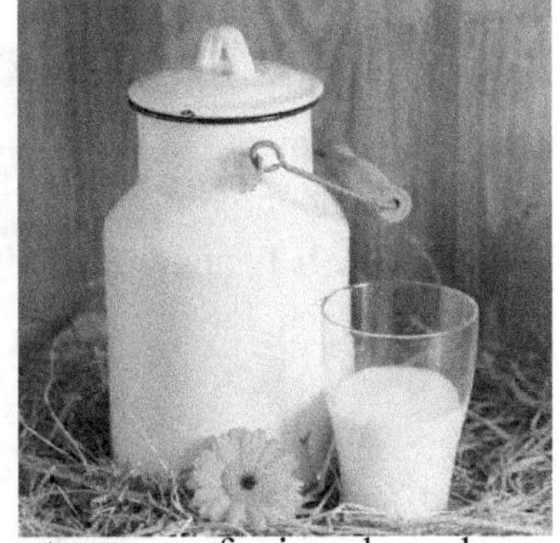

Cow's milk is considered a complete food as it contains almost all the essential nutrients. Whole milk is not only a good source of vitamin D, riboflavin, and vitamin B12, but it is also a source of complete protein and a great source of minerals such as calcium, iodine, and phosphorus.

4. Cheese

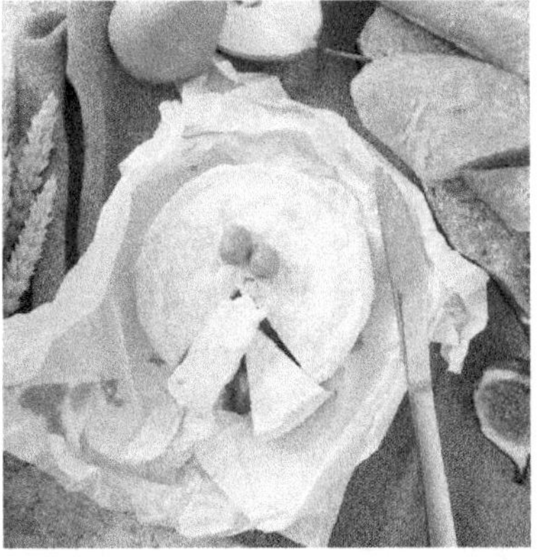

Cheese is high in calcium, protein, and fat, as well as vitamin D. It is also rich in Vitamin A, Riboflavin, and Vitamin B12. For maximum health benefits, choose the right kind of cheese. Cottage cheese, ricotta, and feta cheese are some healthier cheese options you can add to your diet. Although cheddar cheese is high in fat, it is a great source of vitamin D. 100 grams of shredded cheddar cheese contains 6% of your daily value of vitamin D.

5. Yogurt

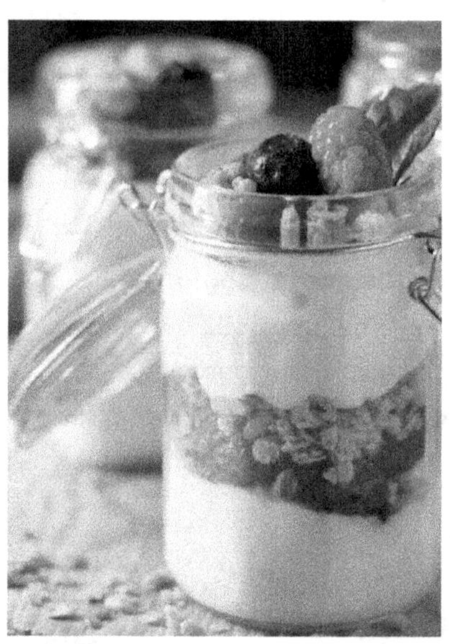

While not the best, curd still provides a decent amount of Vitamin D. It is high in protein and lower in calories than cheese. Additionally, yogurt is a probiotic that promotes gut health. To ensure you meet your daily required vitamin D intake, consider incorporating both yogurt and milk into your diet.

6. Rice Milk

Rice milk is a great alternative to dairy milk. It is made by blending partially boiled rice, usually brown rice, with water. This milk is typically unsweetened and free of saturated fat and cholesterol. It's an ideal option for individuals with allergies who cannot consume soy or almond milk.

7. Butter

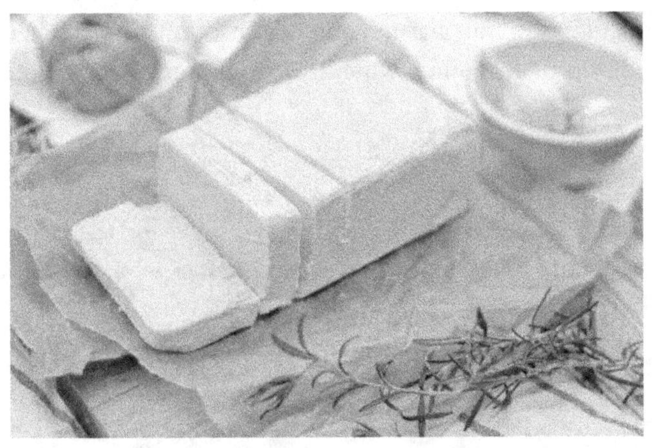

Although butter is often considered unhealthy, when consumed in moderation, it can actually be a nutritious addition to your diet. Butter contains limited vitamin D, and its saturated fat content helps the body absorb antioxidants and vitamin D from other sources. However, consuming butter in moderation is important to avoid potential health issues.

8. Milk Powder

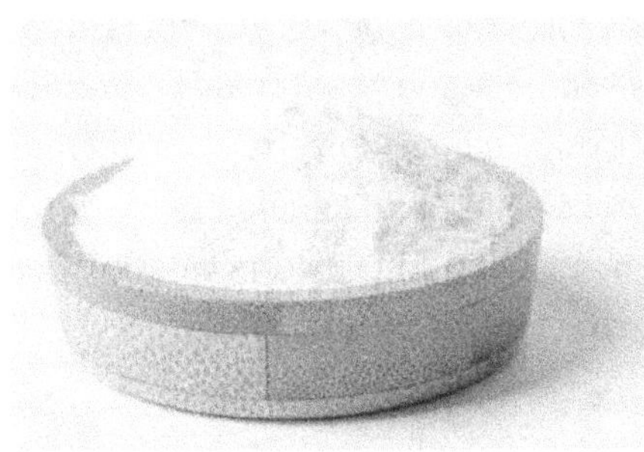

Milk powder is formed by evaporating milk until it becomes dry in order to extend its shelf life. It is packed with Vitamin D and calcium, containing 25.6 IU per cup. Consuming milk powder in moderation is important, as excessive consumption can harm your health due to its oxidized cholesterol content, which can lead to heart-related issues.

9. Sour Cream

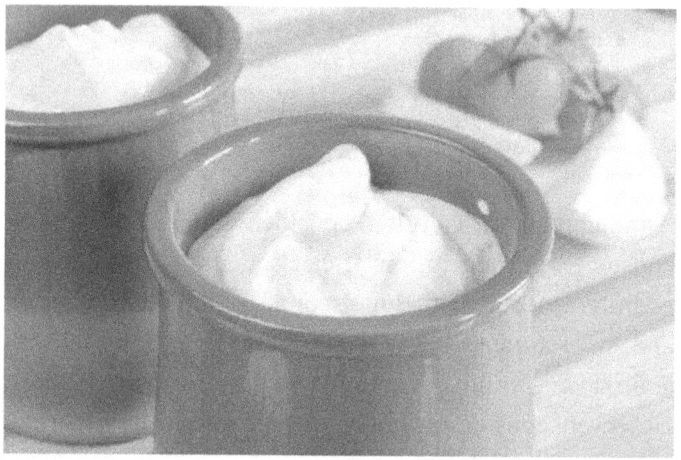

Sour cream often gets a bad reputation when it comes to health, similar to butter. However, it's important to note that sour cream is actually quite nutrient-rich. It contains essential nutrients like protein, vitamin A, potassium, and calcium and can even be a good source of vitamin D for vegetarians. Just one tablespoon of sour cream provides 2 IU of vitamin D and only 28 calories. As with any food, moderation is key, but incorporating sour cream into your diet can be a beneficial choice.

10. Other Not So Natural Sources - Fortified Foods

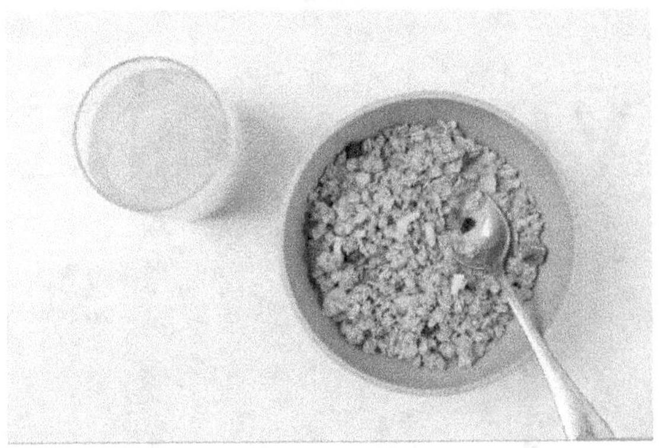

Although orange juice does not contain vitamin D, most orange juices sold in the market are fortified with it. It is important to check the item label to determine the amount of vitamin D added.

Some cereals are fortified with vitamin D, but it may not be sufficient to meet the recommended daily intake. To fulfill your body's vitamin D needs, it is best to have cereals with cow milk. Keep in mind that fortified foods should not be your only source of vitamins, as they are not natural. While it is safe to consume them occasionally, relying solely on fortified foods to meet your body's vitamin needs is not recommended.

Chapter 3
VITAMIN E

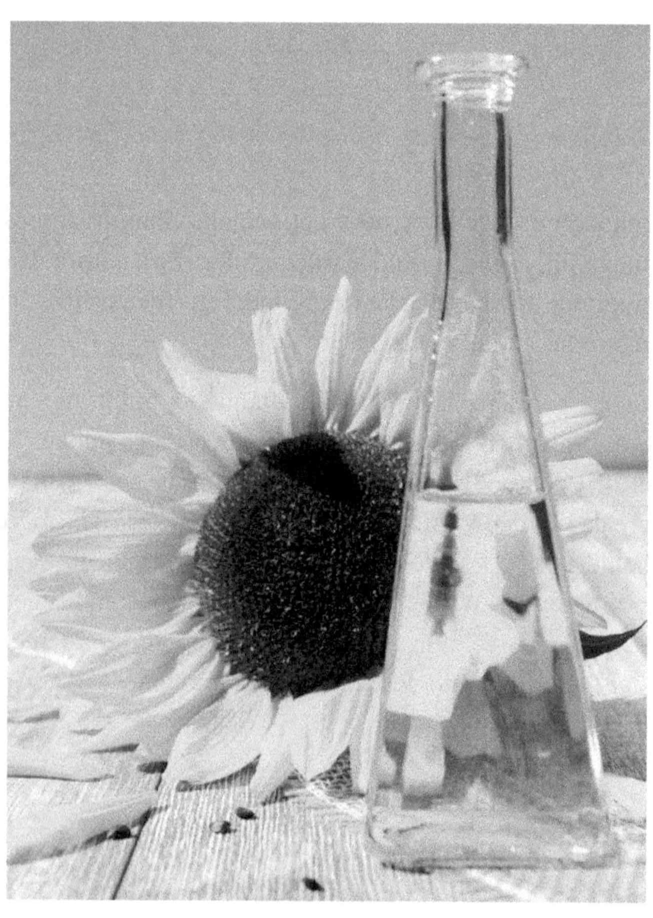

1.

EVERYTHING YOU NEED TO KNOW ABOUT VITAMIN E

The next essential fat-soluble vitamin is Vitamin E. It actually consists of eight different chemical forms - four tocopherols and four tocotrienols. Each form has its own unique antioxidant properties. These tocopherols and tocotrienol forms are as follows:

Tocopherols: alpha-, beta-, gamma-, and delta-tocopherol.

Tocotrienol: alpha-, beta-, gamma-, and delta-tocotrienol

There are eight different forms of vitamin E, each with varying levels of biological activity. However, most of these forms are quickly metabolized by the liver and eliminated from the body. Out of all, only alpha-tocopherol maintains high blood and cellular concentrations, as only this form is re-secreted by the liver through the hepatic alpha-tocopherol transfer protein. This is why vitamin E is commonly referred to as tocopherol or alpha-tocopherol.

Vitamin E is essential for various bodily functions. It acts as an antioxidant that protects cells from harmful free radicals. In the next chapter, we will delve into the details of antioxidants, free radicals, and other crucial roles of Vitamin E. Let's take a look at the recommended daily amount of Vitamin E.

Recommended Intake of Vitamin E

According to the National Institutes of Health Office of Dietary Supplements, in order to fulfill your body's vitamin E (alpha-tocopherol) requirements, the recommended average daily intake amounts are as follows:

Age	Males	Females
0–6 months	4 mg	4 mg
7–12 months	5 mg	5 mg
1–3 years	6 mg	6 mg
4–8 years	7 mg	7 mg
9–13 years	11 mg	11 mg
14+ years	15 mg	15 mg

How common is vitamin E deficiency?

It is rare to experience Vitamin E deficiency due to a diet low in this vitamin. Usually, underlying conditions are the cause. When there is not enough fat present in the digestive tract, the body cannot efficiently absorb fat-soluble vitamins, such as Vitamin E. Individuals who follow extremely low-fat diets may have lower levels of Vitamin E. Additionally, those with fat-malabsorption disorders may also become deficient in Vitamin E. There are certain diseases that prevent fat absorption in the body, which can lead to irregularities in fat absorption or metabolism and ultimately result in Vitamin E deficiency.

Certain health conditions that can lead to vitamin E deficiency are:

• **Crohn's Disease:** Bile acids play a crucial role in facilitating the absorption and transportation of vitamin E. Crohn's disease tends to affect the distal part of the small intestine, known as the terminal ileum. Any damage to the terminal ileum can result in the inadequate absorption of bile acids, leading to vitamin E deficiency.

• **Cystic Fibrosis** is an inherited disorder that results in significant harm to the digestive system and the inability to secrete pancreatic enzymes for absorbing vitamin E.

• **Babies Born prematurely** and weighing less than 1500 grams may have a deficiency in vitamin E.

• **Genetics.**

• **Liver Disease.**

• **Abetalipoproteinemia:** A rare inherited disorder called abetalipoproteinemia results in poor absorption of vitamin E.

• **Ataxia** is another rare inherited disorder caused by a defective or absent alpha-tocopherol transfer protein in the liver, which leads to severe vitamin E deficiency.

What health problems can be caused by Vitamin E deficiency?

If you have a mild deficiency of vitamin E, you can rectify it by incorporating vitamin E-rich foods in your diet instead of taking supplements. However, if your deficiency is due to conditions like Crohn's disease, cystic fibrosis, or other illnesses, your doctor may recommend taking supplements based on your condition. Neglecting vitamin E deficiency may result in severe health issues, including:

Heart Problems: Severe Vitamin E deficiency may lead to the deterioration of muscles, including the heart muscle, and potentially result in cardiac failure.

Hemolytic Anemia: Vitamin E deficiency may lead to the oxidation of red blood cells and ultimately lead to their destruction or hemolysis. In this condition, the body breaks down red blood cells at a faster rate than it can produce them, causing a depletion of red blood cells, resulting in anemia.

Nerve Damage: Vitamin E prevents free radical damage. Nerve cells in the brain are vulnerable to the damaging effects of free radicals. Without enough Vitamin E, nerve cells can die off, which may result in loss of sensation in the extremities (peripheral neuropathy), slurred speech, and loss of reflexes in the legs

Retinopathy of Prematurity (ROP): Retinopathy of Prematurity (ROP) is a condition that affects premature infants, causing the growth of abnormal blood vessels in their eyes. Vitamin E plays a crucial role in protecting cell membranes from oxidation, preventing the oxidation of polyunsaturated fatty acids, which can contribute to the development of ROP. If a premature infant is deficient in vitamin E, they may be at greater risk of developing retinopathy of prematurity

———

While it may not be common to experience a vitamin E deficiency from a low intake of this nutrient in your diet, it is still important to consume enough vitamin E through natural food sources to ensure proper bodily function. Your body may exhibit signs that you are not getting enough vitamin E from your diet. Minor deficiencies can often be corrected through dietary adjustments rather than supplementation. However, it is important to be aware of moderate to severe symptoms of vitamin E deficiency.

Symptoms of Vitamin E Deficiency

If you notice sudden hair loss, unusual dry skin, or more frequent infections, it could be a sign that you are not consuming enough vitamin E in your diet. Other severe symptoms of vitamin E deficiency may include:

- Muscle weakness
- Vision problems
- Difficulty in walking
- Hair fall
- Dry and flaky skin
- Weakened immunity

When should I get tested to rule out a possible Vitamin E deficiency?

If you experience any of the symptoms mentioned above, it is recommended that you undergo a blood test to verify if you have a deficiency in vitamin E.

Am I taking too much Vitamin E?

Consuming too much vitamin E through food is unlikely. It's safe and recommended to have a balanced diet rich in vitamin E from fruits, vegetables, and whole grains. Taking vitamin E supplements without consulting a doctor is not recommended. Excessive intake of vitamin E supplements rather than obtaining it from food sources can lead to hypervitaminosis. Symptoms of excessive vitamin E intake may include:

Fatigue

Diarrhea

Nausea

It's important to be cautious about taking too much vitamin E through supplements, as it can lead to vitamin E toxicity and potentially life-threatening consequences.

To determine any overdose of vitamin E, it is recommended that you consult with your doctor and have a vitamin E test done.

Diagnostic test to determine Vitamin E deficiency or overdose:

The Vitamin E test, also known as the alpha-tocopherol test, is a blood test that measures the level of Vitamin E in your bloodstream. The normal range for Vitamin E levels is:

Adults (18 Years – 150 Years): 5.5 – 17 mg/L

Children (0 – 18 Years): 3.8 – 18.4 mg/L

*Normal ranges may differ slightly between different laboratories.

Do I need to do any preparation before the test?

• This test is taken on an empty stomach, meaning you should not have food or drink for 12-14 hours before the test.

• Do not consume alcohol 24 hours before the test.

• Do not take vitamin supplements 24 hours before the test.

2.

IMPORTANCE OF VITAMIN E

ROLE OF VITAMIN E IN THE BODY

Antioxidant Activity

Vitamin E plays a crucial role as an antioxidant, protecting the body from free radical damage. It is one of the most potent antioxidants available, with the ability to scavenge free radicals and prevent damage to cells. Vitamin E works in two ways to prevent free radical damage. Firstly, it provides a hydrogen atom to unpaired free radicals, breaking the chain reaction and preventing DNA, lipids, and protein damage. Secondly, it limits the production of free radicals altogether. Free radicals are highly reactive and can cause damage to cell structures. ROS (reactive oxygen species) are formed as a by-product of the oxidation of dietary fats to produce energy in the body. In lesser amounts, ROS helps to kill invading pathogens and regulate normal physiological functions at the cellular level. However, excessive ROS formation can lead to oxidative stress and result in various diseases. Vitamin E, a fat-soluble antioxidant, helps prevent ROS production and thus protects against chronic diseases caused by free radicals.

Anti-Inflammatory Action

Inflammation is a defense mechanism used by the immune system to protect the body against foreign attackers, such as viruses and bacteria. Although inflammation is a beneficial process, it can sometimes harm the body. In some cases, the immune system mistakenly attacks the body's own cells, leading to harmful inflammation. This can result in autoimmune diseases like rheumatoid arthritis, osteoporosis, psoriasis, inflammatory bowel diseases, and type 1 diabetes. To reduce inflammation in the body, certain substances interfere with the chemical reactions that cause it. These substances are called anti-inflammatory agents. Vitamin E is one such agent that plays an important role in anti-inflammatory processes. COX-2 enzymes produce prostaglandins that promote pain and inflammation. Vitamin E inhibits these inflammation-causing COX-2 enzymes. Vitamin E also suppresses the production of pro-inflammatory cytokines. Free radicals activate transcription factor NFκB, which leads to the production of inflammation-causing cytokines. Vitamin E neutralizes free radicals before they can activate NFκB, suppressing cytokine production and reducing inflammation.

Inhibits Platelet Aggregation

Platelets play a crucial role in hemostasis and thrombosis, which are processes related to blood clotting. Hemostasis is the initial stage of clotting, where the blood transforms from a liquid state to a gel-like state to prevent further bleeding. While blood clotting is vital in wound healing, it can be harmful if it occurs inside blood vessels. Thrombosis is the medical term for blood clot formation within a blood vessel. This can impede blood flow through the circulatory system, leading to health complications like heart attacks or strokes. Alpha-tocopherol can help inhibit protein kinase C activity, which is an enzyme involved in platelet secretion and aggregation.

Vitamin E has another way of preventing platelet aggregation: by increasing the production of vasodilators. Prostacyclin, a member of the prostaglandin family, is a powerful inhibitor of platelet activation and a vasodilator. Vitamin E, specifically D-alpha-tocopherol, triggers the release of prostacyclin from the endothelium cells lining the inside of blood vessels. This, in turn, dilates blood vessels and prevents platelet aggregation. This effect is due to vitamin E having an opposing effect on the two key regulatory enzymes in prostacyclin biosynthesis, which results in a net increase in the production of vasodilator prostacyclin in endothelial cells.

Role in Immune Enhancement

Direct Effect:

Vitamin E is found in higher levels in immune cells compared to other cells in the body. It's actually one of the most effective nutrients when it comes to regulating immune function. Vitamin E has the ability to protect the polyunsaturated fatty acids (PUFAs) in the cell membrane from oxidative damage. Immune cells are highly influenced by cell membrane composition and structure as their membranes are a primary site for translating external signals. By preventing oxidation and cell membrane damage, Vitamin E helps maintain membrane integrity and signal transduction, which ultimately affects the function of immune cells.

Indirect Effect:

T cells are the white blood cells of the immune system that has a central role in the immune response to infection. They carry out their function either as killer cells that kill cells infected with a virus and cancer cells or as helper cells, aiding B cells in producing antibodies. When T cells are not functioning properly, it can lead to a higher risk of contracting infectious diseases and a weaker response to immunization.

Vitamin E can regulate the immune system's T cells by modulating inflammation-causing cytokines and prostaglandin E2 (PGE2). PGE2 is a pro-inflammatory prostaglandin that suppresses T-cell response by inhibiting T-cell proliferation and Interleukin-2 (IL-2) production. However, Vitamin E can inhibit prostaglandin E2 production by suppressing cyclooxygenase 2 (COX2) enzyme activity that converts arachidonic acid to prostaglandins. This results in an increase in the cell division and Interleukin-2-producing capacity of naïve T cells, which in turn increases the percentage of T cells. IL-2, which is responsible for activating T cells, has the potential to kill cancerous cells and reduce the size of tumors wherever they develop in the body.

Top 10 Most Significant Health Benefits of Vitamin E

1. Prevent Coronary Heart Disease

When cholesterol builds up in the walls of arteries that supply blood to the heart, it can block blood flow and cause coronary heart disease. This build-up can cause the arteries to narrow over time. This process is known as atherosclerosis, and the cholesterol deposits are called atheroma. A crucial factor in atherosclerosis is low-density lipoprotein (LDL) cholesterol. Vitamin E can effectively prevent or delay coronary heart disease by inhibiting the oxidation of LDL cholesterol. Additionally, vitamin E can help prevent blood clots that may lead to a heart attack by inhibiting platelet aggregation.

2. Prevent Cancer

Vitamin E plays an important role in protecting cell integrity from harmful free radicals, which can contribute to the development of cancer. A deficiency of vitamin E can increase the risk of cancer. Vitamin E prevents prostate cancer in men who are at high risk of prostate cancer. Consuming foods rich in vitamin E can greatly decrease the likelihood of developing advanced prostate cancer, particularly for individuals who have quit smoking.

Nitrosamines, which are metabolites of nicotine found in cigarette smoke, are major cancer-causing agents. These nitrosamines can generate free radicals that damage the DNA. Additionally, nitrosamines can also be created from nitrate and nitrite, which are added to processed meat to keep it fresh for longer. When processed meat is cooked at high temperatures, the protein in it reacts with nitrates to create an ideal environment for the formation of nitrosamines, which are known to be carcinogenic. Vitamin E can help block the formation of these cancer-causing nitrosamines and protect against various types of cancer by enhancing immune function.

You may be curious as to why nitrates are considered carcinogenic, even though nitrates in beetroot can help lower blood pressure and prevent heart disease (as specified in the book **Eat to Prevent and Control Disease**). The reason is that vegetables, like beetroot, are not high in protein and are rarely cooked at high temperatures. Additionally, vegetables contain protective elements such as vitamin C, fiber, and polyphenols, all of which have been shown to decrease the formation of nitrosamines. These factors contribute to the health benefits of beetroot and other vegetables despite the presence of nitrates.

3. Prevent Eyes Disorder

As you age, you may experience age-related eye problems such as Age-related macular degeneration (AMD) and cataracts. These issues are the most common causes of vision loss among older individuals. Your retina and macula are essential components of your eye that enable clear and central vision. Macular degeneration occurs when the macula degrades, which typically happens as you age, hence the term age-related macular degeneration. Cataracts, on the other hand, occur when protein accumulates in the lens of your eye, causing cloudy vision. Oxidative stress caused by free radicals can harm the macula and protein within the eye. Vitamin E functions as an antioxidant and can prevent these types of damage to the eyes. Numerous studies have shown that vitamin E obtained through a healthy diet is highly effective in preventing eye disorders, although taking vitamin E supplements has not yielded positive results.

4. Prevent Influenza

Influenza is a type of viral infection that affects your respiratory system, including your lungs, nose, and throat. While vitamin E does not offer specific antiviral benefits, its antioxidant properties can help protect your lungs and prevent oxidative damage caused by influenza.

Severe influenza can cause damage to the lungs by triggering viral replication and inflammation, which generates free radicals that harm the cellular membranes of blood vessels. These excess free radicals cause the oxidation of unsaturated fats in cell membranes. Since vitamin E is fat-soluble, it accumulates in fat membranes and exerts antioxidant action there. It reacts with unpaired electrons of free radicals and can prevent them from reacting with adjacent fatty acid side chains. Due to its effectiveness in preventing oxidative damage through its free-radical scavenging activity, vitamin E is the most efficient antioxidant for influenza virus infection.

5. Prevent Asthma

Research shows that individuals with asthma often have lower levels of vitamin E, and vitamin E deficiency is linked with the severity of asthma symptoms. Vitamin E can reduce inflammation and act as an antioxidant, which could be beneficial for those with asthma. However, there have been conflicting results from different studies on the effects of vitamin E supplements on asthma. Some studies suggest that high levels of alpha-tocopherol, a major form of vitamin E, could lead to a decrease in lung function, whereas other studies dispute this finding and instead propose that alpha-tocopherol can actually improve lung function, while gamma-tocopherol might reduce it.

Asthmatics have low levels of vitamin E, which is essential in reducing inflammation. Therefore, increasing dietary intake of vitamin E may help prevent or control allergic diseases and asthma. Furthermore, vitamin E has been shown to reduce levels of mucins, which affect the stickiness of mucus. This is particularly important as people with asthma often have elevated levels of mucins.

6. Prevent Osteoporosis

Osteoporosis is a bone disease characterized by low bone mass and an increased risk of fractures. Normally, your body constantly replaces bone tissue to keep your bones healthy. However, in osteoporosis, new bone is not formed as old bone is removed, resulting in bone loss. This loss of bone mass weakens the bones, making them more susceptible to fractures. Chronic inflammation is the primary cause of osteoporosis. When inflammation occurs near the bones, it often increases bone resorption, degrading the bone without any subsequent coupling to new bone formation. Older people are particularly prone to osteoporosis, as they tend to produce more pro-inflammatory cytokines as they age.

Inflammation is triggered when free radicals activate transcription factor NFκB, which leads to the production of the cytokines interleukin-1 and interleukin-6. These pro-inflammatory cytokines cause bone resorption. Vitamin E can help prevent osteoporosis by scavenging and neutralizing free radicals before they can activate transcription factor NFκB. Vitamin E also enhances the internal antioxidative enzymes within the bone, which further help prevent the activation of NFκB.

In addition, vitamin E acts as an anti-inflammatory agent to safeguard bones from degradation. Vitamin E decreases the production of prostaglandins, the culprits behind inflammation. It hinders the activity of COX-2 enzymes responsible for the production of prostaglandins.

7. Prevent Alzheimer's Disease and Other Neurodegenerative Diseases

Neurodegenerative diseases are irreversible conditions that primarily affect nerve cells in the human brain. This happens when nerve cells lose their structure or function, leading to cell death. Over time, free radical damage to nerve cells contributes to the development of these diseases. In particular, oxidative stress is a major player in Alzheimer's disease and is involved in its initiation and progression. The brain is composed of 60% fat and consumes 20% of the total oxygen in the body. Lipid peroxidation and protein oxidation in the brain can trigger Alzheimer's disease. Vitamin E can reduce oxidative stress and improve memory and cognitive deficits.

Research shows that consuming more vitamin E through a balanced diet, rather than relying on high-dose supplements, is linked to a lower risk of neurodegenerative diseases. You may significantly reduce your chances of developing neurodegenerative conditions by incorporating vitamin E-rich foods into your diet, along with other potent antioxidants like carotenoids and vitamin C.

8. Enhance Skin Health

Exposure to ultraviolet rays from sunlight, dust, air pollution, and smoke can cause free radicals to form in your skin cells, leading to brown spots, wrinkles, and premature aging. Applying vitamin E oil topically may help reverse this damage by acting as a free-radical scavenger. Additionally, using vitamin E and vitamin C together can provide even greater protection against UV rays, as vitamin C enhances vitamin E's antioxidant action and produces synergistic results.

9. Boost Hair Health

Vitamin E is essential in maintaining your scalp health. Vitamin E is an antioxidant that helps protect the cellular membrane of your hair follicles from damage-causing free radicals. This action ensures that oxygen and nutrient-rich blood are delivered to your hair, which helps moisturize and hydrate dry and brittle hair. This, in turn, helps strengthen the hair follicles and prevents hair loss.

Additionally, vitamin E has anti-inflammatory properties that help reduce inflammation that can cause hair follicle cells to break down. This helps prevent hair loss and promotes healthy and strong hair growth.

Vitamin E also helps prevent premature graying of hair and split ends. Free radicals can damage cells and accelerate the aging process, but vitamin E helps prevent the depletion of cells, which helps combat the premature graying of hair. Moreover, oxidative damage to the hair follicles can cause split ends, but applying vitamin E oil topically can help seal them and prevent further splits.

10. Premenstrual Syndrome (PMS)

Approximately 90% of women experience premenstrual syndrome (PMS) symptoms, such as pain, mood swings, stress, bloating, fatigue, and other physical and emotional changes, one to two weeks before their period begins. These symptoms can adversely affect the quality of life and daily work. Fortunately, antioxidant vitamin E can help alleviate PMS symptoms by reducing lipid oxidation and inhibiting the release of arachidonic acid and its conversion to pain-producing prostaglandins. This makes vitamin E significant in reducing the severity and duration of menstrual cramps. Additionally, vitamin E can significantly reduce irritability, stress, and other mood symptoms associated with PMS.

3.

10 RICHEST FOOD SOURCES OF VITAMIN E

NUTS & SEEDS

Nuts and seeds are the primary sources of vitamin E due to their abundance of healthy fats and numerous health benefits. Incorporating these into your diet is a wise investment in your overall health. Consuming a handful of mixed nuts and seeds daily can reduce your risk of chronic diseases. However, during summer, limiting consumption to four times a week is advised, as nuts and seeds can generate heat in the body and potentially cause mouth ulcers.

While most dry fruits contain vitamin E, some are richer sources than others. Let's take a look at the ones with the highest vitamin E content:

1. Sunflower Seeds

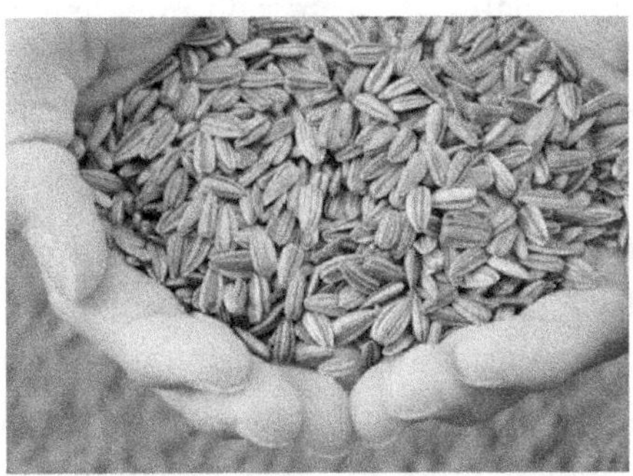

Sunflower seeds are a rich source of vitamin E. Just a handful (about 30 grams) of dry roasted sunflower seeds contain 49% of your daily recommended intake of vitamin E. These seeds also contain other beneficial nutrients like potassium, magnesium, fiber, and zinc that can help lower the risk of developing high blood pressure, diabetes, and heart disease. Additionally, the vitamin E, flavonoids, and plant compounds in sunflower seeds can help reduce chronic inflammation.

However, if you suffer from arthritis, it's best to avoid consuming excessive amounts of sunflower seeds because sunflower seeds contain high levels of omega-6 fats, which can aggravate your arthritis symptoms. It's important to consume omega-6 fatty acids in moderation.

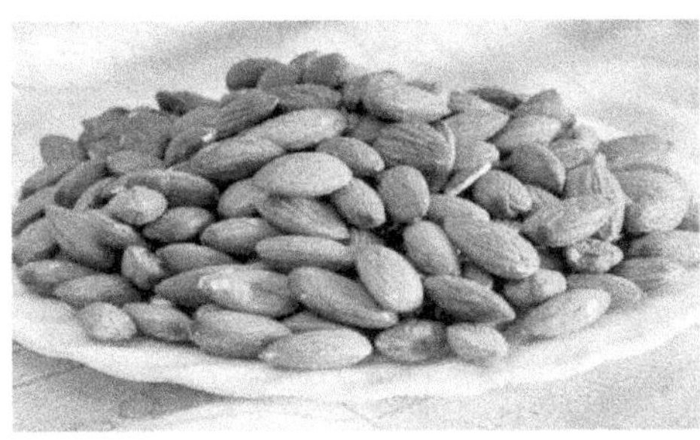

2. Almonds

Almonds are not only delicious but also nutritious. They contain a variety of healthy components such as vitamin E, fiber, monounsaturated fats, and protein. Additionally, they are rich in essential minerals like magnesium, iron, calcium, copper, and zinc. Eating a handful of dry roasted almonds (around 23 kernels) can provide you with 45% of your recommended daily vitamin E intake. Almonds are a great snack option because they are low in carbohydrates and high in protein. The protein in almonds slows down digestion and makes you feel fuller for longer, aiding in weight loss by reducing hunger. Moreover, eating almonds can help lower the risk of type 2 diabetes and hypertension, as they are high in magnesium. Vitamin E in almond oil can also be beneficial for your skin, healing sun damage and giving you a smooth and glowing complexion. And for those looking to improve hair growth, massaging your scalp with almond oil can provide numerous health benefits.

For optimum health benefits, consider consuming soaked almonds. The skin of almonds contains phytic acid that can hinder the absorption of vital minerals like iron, magnesium, zinc, copper, and calcium. Soaking almonds overnight helps to reduce their phytic acid levels, thereby enhancing the absorption of these essential minerals.

3. Peanuts

Peanuts are rich in protein, fiber, potassium, Vitamin E, and healthy fats. Just a handful (30 gm) of dry roasted peanuts can provide you with 15% of your daily recommended vitamin E intake. Peanuts are great for maintaining a healthy heart as they help lower cholesterol levels and prevent blood clots in the arteries, 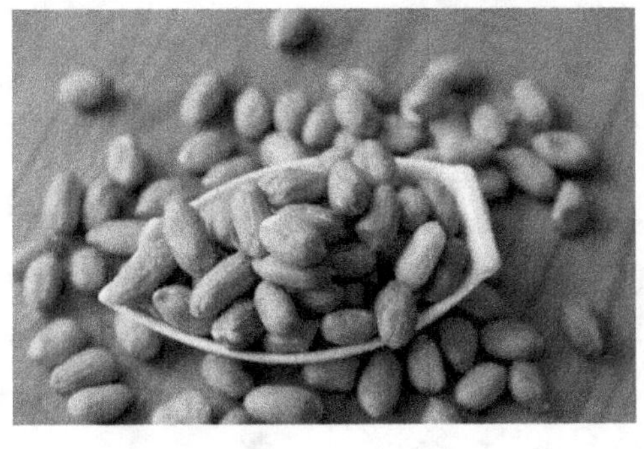 which can reduce your risk of heart attack or stroke. For those with diabetes, peanuts make a perfect snack as they have a low glycemic index, which means they are slowly digested and cause a slower rise in blood sugar levels. Additionally, the manganese present in peanuts can improve glucose metabolism and increase insulin secretion.

It is recommended that you limit your daily peanut consumption to between 30 and 60 grams. While peanuts contain healthy unsaturated fats, they are also high in calories and saturated fats. To maintain normal cholesterol levels, it is important to keep your consumption of saturated fats to no more than 10% of your daily total fat intake.

VEGETABLE OILS

Adding vegetable oil to your diet is one of the easiest ways to get vitamin E, which is also a great source of healthy fats like polyunsaturated and monounsaturated fats. To get the maximum health benefits, it is important to avoid heating these oils at very high temperatures (>200 °C) and to avoid reusing the same oil multiple times. When deep frying, temperatures around 180 °C are required. However, high temperatures can cause the oil to break down and change its chemical structure, forming harmful compounds that can be absorbed by your fried food and increase the risk of cancer. To prevent this, keep the flame at medium or medium-high, and reduce it to low if you see smoke. Discard any remaining oil and avoid reusing it.

4. Wheat Germ Oil

Vitamin E is abundant in wheat germ oil. Just one tablespoon of this oil contains 135% of the daily recommended value of this important nutrient. Wheat germ oil is extracted from the germ, which is the most nutritious part of the wheat kernel. While it may have a distinct taste that some people don't find pleasant, it is incredibly nutritious. It's also rich in octacosanol, which has been shown to have anti-parkinsonism effects and can improve the way your body uses oxygen to boost muscular energy. Wheat germ oil's high vitamin E content makes it a superfood for your skin and hair. Its ability to scavenge free radicals helps prevent wrinkles and other signs of aging while also promoting good scalp health and stimulating healthy hair growth.

To extend the shelf life of your wheat germ oil, it's important to store it properly. Due to its high unsaturated fat content, it can quickly become rancid when exposed to oxygen in the air. Therefore, keeping it in an airtight container in a cool and dark location is recommended. This will help maintain the quality and freshness of the oil for a longer period of time.

5. Sunflower Oil

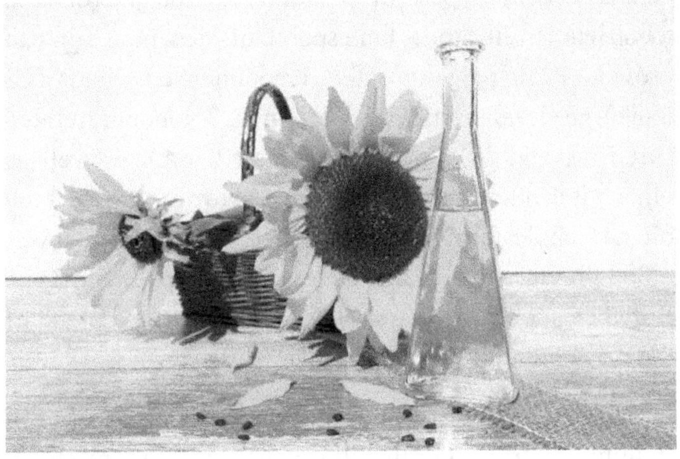

Sunflower oil is one of the best sources of vitamin E and can help promote heart health. Just one tablespoon of sunflower oil contains 47% of the daily recommended value of Vitamin E. The monounsaturated fat (oleic acid) found in sunflower oil is beneficial for heart health. Vitamin E helps prevent cholesterol from oxidizing and keeps blood vessels intact while also preventing clots from forming. Additionally, the high linoleic acid content found in sunflower oil can also provide cardiovascular benefits and reduce the risk of heart disease. However, it's important to consume sunflower oil in moderation, as it is high in omega-6 fats, and too much consumption can lead to inflammation.

6. Rice Bran Oil

In recent years, the popularity of rice bran oil has increased because of its potential health advantages. It contains both types of vitamin E, tocopherol and tocotrienols. Just one tablespoon of rice bran oil can provide 32% of your daily recommended vitamin E intake. It is also rich in vitamin K, monounsaturated (MUFA), and polyunsaturated fats (PUFA), as well as other vital nutrients. Studies have shown that rice bran oil has cholesterol-lowering effects. It can help lower blood pressure and is also beneficial for those with Type II diabetes. For maximum health benefits, use a blend of 80% rice bran oil with 20% sesame oil.

In addition, using rice bran oil for oil pulling can aid in fighting bad breath (halitosis). Simply take a tablespoon (15 ml) of oil into your mouth and swish it around for 10 minutes before spitting it out. Then, rinse your mouth with a glass of water for 1 minute.

Other notable oils rich in vitamin E are cottonseed oil (35% of DV), safflower oil (31% of DV), corn oil (13% of DV), and soybean oil (7% of DV).

VEGETABLES

While vegetables and fruits may not be the most abundant sources of vitamin E, they do contain some amount of this essential nutrient. Moreover, they are packed with other important nutrients and vitamins. To ensure that you meet your daily recommended intake of all vitamins, it is best to follow a balanced diet that includes grains, legumes, healthy oils, nuts, and seeds, as well as fruits and vegetables. Relying solely on one food source for your vitamin intake can deprive you of the health benefits that come from other foods.

7. Spinach

Spinach is considered a superfood due to its abundance of essential nutrients and health benefits. It 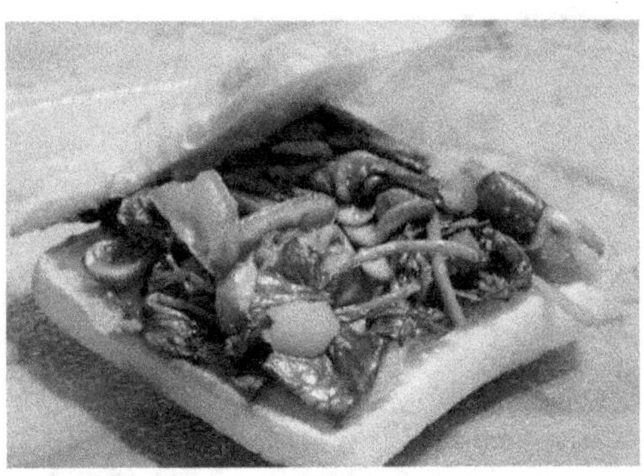 contains high potassium, magnesium, calcium, iron, and vitamins A, K, and E levels. In fact, just half a cup of boiled spinach provides 13% of the daily recommended intake of vitamin E. Additionally, spinach is known for its anti-inflammatory and anti-oxidative properties, which can help reduce the risk of high blood pressure. Studies have also found that increased consumption of spinach may lower the risk of asthma in children, likely due to its high content of beta-carotene and vitamin E, both of which have been shown to play a role in reducing airway inflammation.

Those with kidney problems should limit their consumption of spinach as consuming it in excess may cause kidney stones. Additionally, if you are taking blood-thinning medication, it is important to consult with your doctor and pharmacist to determine the appropriate daily intake of spinach, as it may reduce the effectiveness of your medication.

8. Broccoli

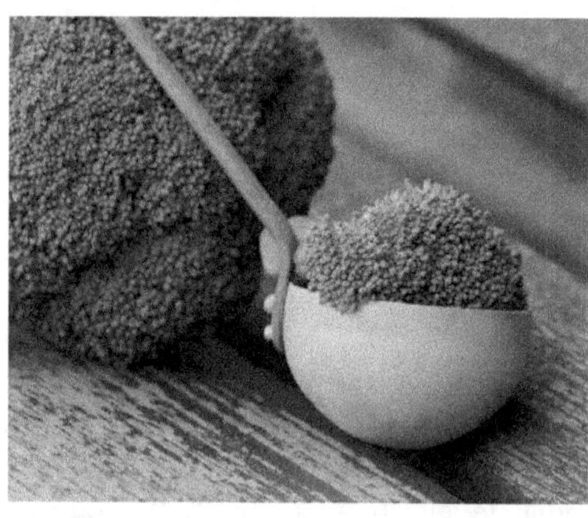

Do you know broccoli leaves have more antioxidants than the florets and stems? Broccoli is jam-packed with antioxidants, including vitamins E, C, and A, which help to strengthen the immune system and prevent damage to cells caused by free radicals. Plus, it's rich in sulforaphane, a powerful compound that can help prevent cancer cell formation and lower blood sugar levels. Half a cup of boiled broccoli can provide 7% of your daily recommended vitamin E intake.

Other notable vitamin E-rich vegetables are red bell peppers, pumpkin, and tomatoes.

FRUITS

9. Avocado

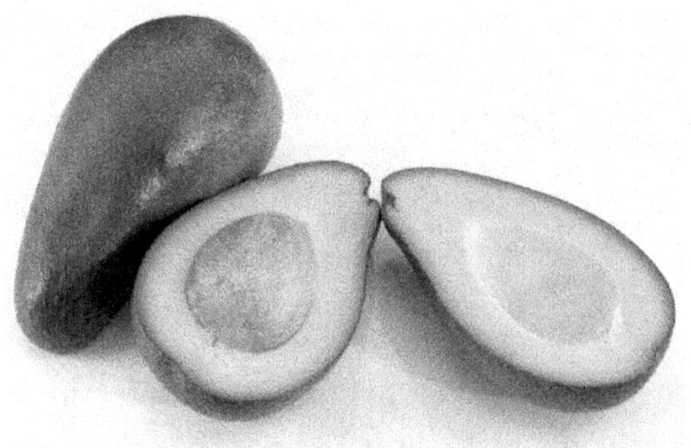

Avocado has a moderate amount of vitamin E. Half of an avocado (around 100 grams) contains 14% of the daily value of vitamin E, making it a healthy addition to your diet. While avocado has a high-fat content of about 75%, it's important to note that it's mostly heart-healthy monounsaturated fat, such as oleic acid. The remaining fat is saturated fat. Interestingly, avocados contain more potassium than bananas. Consuming avocados in moderation can help protect you against cardiovascular diseases. Avocados' high monounsaturated fat content can help lower your LDL cholesterol levels (bad cholesterol), while vitamin E can prevent cholesterol deposition by preventing blood clots and oxidative damage. Additionally, potassium can help keep your blood pressure within normal limits and reduce your heart disease and stroke risk.

10 Kiwi

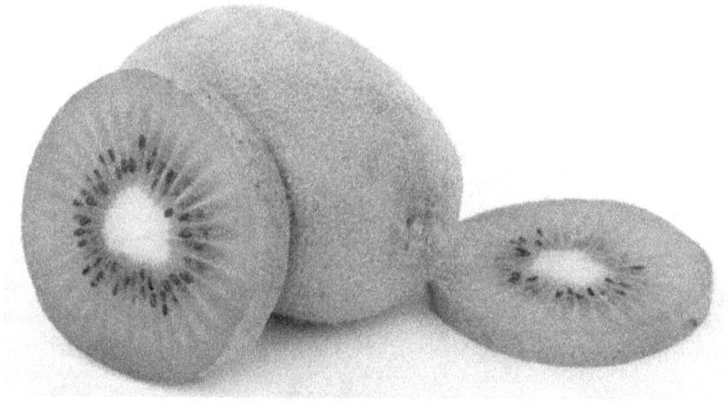

Kiwis are among the richest sources of vitamin C and have a generous amount of antioxidant vitamin E, which are antioxidants that can help boost your immunity and prevent chronic inflammatory diseases. Just one medium green kiwi can provide 7% of your daily requirement of vitamin E. These antioxidants work by killing free radicals before they can cause damage to your cells. Kiwis are also rich in potassium, which helps to promote blood vessel relaxation and lower blood pressure. Plus, the fiber in kiwis can help prevent constipation and keep your cholesterol levels in check.

Other notable fruits rich in vitamin E are mango and blackberry.

Effect of Cooking Temperature on Vitamin E:

Vitamin E in Green Vegetables

Boiling or blanching your green leafy vegetables can increase their vitamin E content. This is because cooking breaks down the cell walls of plants, which releases vitamin E from the lipids. However, cutting or mixing vegetables can activate oxidizing enzymes that cause vitamin E loss. To prevent this, it's best to use heat treatment, which deactivates these enzymes and preserves the vitamin E content. Therefore, it's best to boil or blanch green vegetables instead of eating them raw to get maximum vitamin E.

Vitamin E in Oils

When cooking with Vitamin E, it's important to be mindful of the temperature and cooking time. While Vitamin E is generally stable in heat, high-heat cooking methods like frying can cause a loss of this important nutrient. Studies have shown that heating oil at 210 °C or more can result in a loss of 6.38% of Vitamin E. Additionally, cooking at very high temperatures (over 250 °C) for longer periods of time can reduce the Vitamin E content by up to 20%. To ensure you're getting the most out of Vitamin E-rich foods like almonds and cooking oils, it's best to avoid deep frying or baking at high temperatures (over 200 °C) and cook them for shorter periods of time.

Chapter 4

VITAMIN K

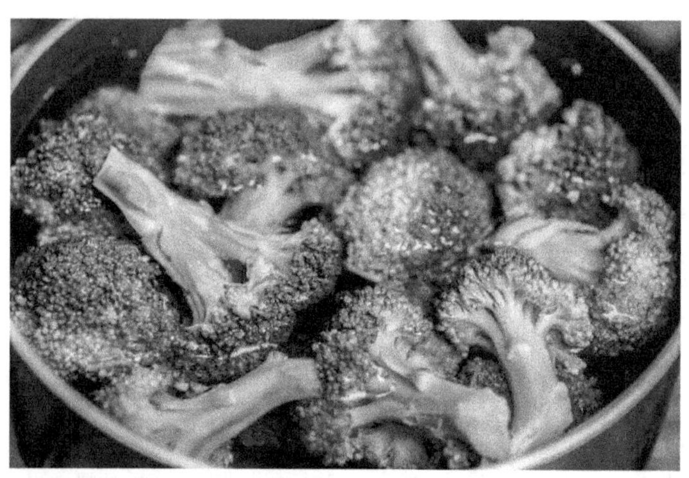

1.

EVERYTHING YOU NEED TO KNOW ABOUT VITAMIN K

Vitamin K is an essential fat-soluble vitamin that your body needs to produce crucial proteins such as prothrombin. This protein plays a vital role in blood clotting and wound healing. Additionally, Vitamin K is crucial for the production of osteocalcin and Matrix Gla-protein, which are necessary for maintaining healthy bones.

Forms of Vitamin K

Vitamin K has two natural forms and one synthetic form

Vitamin K1: Phylloquinone (Natural)

Vitamin K2: Menaquinone (Natural)

Vitamin K3: Menadione (Synthetic)

Vitamin K1 (Phylloquinone)

The primary source of dietary vitamin K is phylloquinone (K1). This essential nutrient is synthesized by plants and is mostly present in green leafy vegetables. Approximately 90% of the total vitamin K in your diet comes from Vitamin K1. The recommended Adequate Intakes (AI) for vitamin K are solely based on phylloquinone.

Vitamin K2 (Menaquinone)

Vitamin K2, or menaquinone, is produced by bacteria and can be found in small amounts in fermented foods, milk, and butter. There are different types of menaquinones, ranging from MK-4 to MK-13, based on the length of their side chain. The most well-researched types of menaquinones are MK-4, MK-7, and MK-9. Interestingly, the body can also convert phylloquinone (K1) into Menaquinone MK-4. Your gut bacteria can produce almost all types of menaquinones, which can fulfill some of the body's vitamin K needs, but not all.

Vitamin K3 (Menadione)

Menadione is a synthetic manmade form of vitamin K. It is converted into menaquinone in the liver and was once used as a dietary supplement. However, it has since been banned by the FDA due to its harmful side effects. These include the destruction of red blood cells (hemolytic anemia) and damage to the liver. Large doses of menadione have also been linked to brain damage. As a result, its use has been discontinued.

How does Vitamin K work in the Body?

When you consume a meal that is rich in vitamin K, the vitamin is absorbed into mixed micelles that consist of bile salts and pancreatic enzymes. These micelles are then absorbed in the small intestine and transported to the liver. Vitamin K1 is transported by triglyceride-rich lipoproteins (TRL), while vitamin K2 is mainly transported by low-density lipoproteins (LDL) to various tissues in the body. Vitamin K is present in many parts of the body, including the liver, brain, bones, heart, and pancreas.

Phylloquinone, the plant form of vitamin K, is not well absorbed by the body. Only 30% to 40% of the total consumption actually remains in the body to provide health benefits. The rest is metabolized and excreted, with 20% leaving through urine and 40% to 50% through feces. This is why Vitamin K toxicity is rare, even with excessive consumption, due to the low absorption rate. However, consuming healthy fats with vitamin K can greatly increase its absorption.

How much Vitamin K do I need?

There isn't sufficient evidence available to establish Recommended Dietary Allowance (RDA) for vitamin K. Therefore, the Food and Nutrition Board (FNB) has established Adequate Intake (AI) to ensure nutritional adequacy in the healthy population.

Age	Male	Female
Birth to 6 months	2.0 mcg	2.0 mcg
7–12 months	2.5 mcg	2.5 mcg
1–3 years	30 mcg	30 mcg
4–8 years	55 mcg	55 mcg
9–13 years	60 mcg	60 mcg
14–18 years	75 mcg	75 mcg
19+ years	120 mcg	90 mcg

Deficiency in Vitamin K

Vitamin K deficiency can lead to excessive bleeding as it is necessary for the formation of blood clots. Although it is rare for a poor diet to cause a deficiency, individuals who take blood-thinning medication like warfarin, those with a disease that affects the absorption of Vitamin K, those who have undergone weight loss surgery, and newborns are at risk of deficiency. Newborns, in particular, require a Vitamin K injection at birth to prevent deficiency. Here are more details:

Vitamin K Shots for Newborns

All newborns must receive vitamin K shots shortly after birth to prevent excessive bleeding, which may result in hemorrhagic disease of the newborn (HDN). According to the Centers for Disease Control and Prevention (CDC), newborns who do not receive the vitamin K shot are 81 times more likely to experience severe bleeding than those who do get the shot.

There are many reasons why newborns are prone to vitamin K deficiency:

- Babies aren't born with enough Vitamin K in their body.
- Vitamin K doesn't cross the placenta well.
- Mother's milk has very low levels of Vitamin K.
- Babies have insufficient gut bacteria to produce vitamin K2.
- The liver of babies is not able to efficiently utilize vitamin K.

Lactating mothers should ensure they consume sufficient amounts of vitamin K through diet or by taking prescribed multivitamins to maintain healthy levels of vitamin K in the baby for up to six months or until the baby obtains it from another source.

While it is uncommon for adults to experience vitamin K deficiency, it is still possible that you may have low levels of this essential nutrient. Signs of a deficiency may include bleeding in different areas of the body or prolonged bleeding after a cut. To address this issue, you can increase your consumption of foods rich in vitamin K. Below are some symptoms that may indicate low levels or deficiency of vitamin K.

Signs and Symptoms of Vitamin K Deficiency

• Nosebleeds

• Bleeding gum

• Easy bruising

• Uncontrolled bleeding from wounds.

• Heavy period flow.

• Bleeding from the gastrointestinal (GI) tract.

• Blood in the urine

• Blood in the stool.

• Blackish stool.

Reasons/Risk Factors for Vitamin K Deficiency

Vitamin K deficiency is not only caused by inadequate intake but also by other risk factors and health conditions.

Long-Term Antibiotic Treatment: Antibiotics are effective in eliminating harmful bacteria, but they can also eliminate vitamin K-synthesizing bacterial flora. Prolonged antibiotic use can lead to a deficiency in vitamin K due to the loss of these bacteria. As a result, it is common for doctors to prescribe multivitamins alongside antibiotics to prevent this deficiency.

Fat Malabsorption: In this condition, fat from your food is not absorbed in your small intestine and passes through your colon unabsorbed, resulting in fatty stools. This can prevent important fat-soluble vitamins, such as vitamin K, from being absorbed by your body, leading to vitamin K deficiency.

Liver Disease: People with liver cirrhosis and those with coexisting biliary disease have reduced bile production and bile flow, which leads to a decreased amount of biliary salts. This decreases the absorption of fat-soluble vitamins, including vitamin K.

Certain Disease Conditions: Certain disease conditions, such as Crohn's disease, can cause fat malabsorption that results in vitamin K deficiency.

Short Bowel Syndrome: A condition that affects people who've had part of the small intestine removed, due to which the body is unable to effectively absorb nutrients from the foods, resulting in vitamin K deficiency.

Anti-Coagulation Medicines: Anticoagulants or anti-clotting drugs, which are commonly known as blood thinners, are vitamin K antagonists that prevent blood clotting. They interfere in the blood clotting process by preventing the formation or working of certain clotting factors. Excessive use of anticoagulants can result in vitamin K deficiency.

How is Vitamin K deficiency diagnosed?

If you experience frequent bruising or excessive bleeding from a cut, or unexpected bleeding, your doctor may ask you to be tested for vitamin K deficiency.

To detect vitamin K deficiency, a prothrombin time (PT) test is used. Prothrombin protein (clotting factor 2) is one of the 13 clotting (coagulation) factors that help blood to clot. This test is the measurement of the time it takes for blood to clot. If the prothrombin time is prolonged, it could indicate low vitamin K levels in the body. To confirm a vitamin K deficiency, oral vitamin K supplements or injections may be administered. If the prothrombin time returns to normal after this treatment, it is confirmed that you have vitamin K deficiency.

Reference range: 11 to 13.5 seconds

This particular blood test is also known as PT/INR or Protime INR. INR stands for international normalized ratio and is derived from the prothrombin time and ensures that the outcome is consistent across different laboratories. The World Health Organization (WHO) has established a method for calculating INR:

INR = Patient PT ÷ Control PT

Note: Under certain conditions, false reports of vitamin K deficiency may occur. Taking blood-thinning medications like warfarin can cause an increase in prothrombin time, which can misleadingly indicate a vitamin K deficiency. To avoid inaccurate results, inform your doctor of any current health conditions and medications before undergoing a vitamin K deficiency test.

Effect of Cooking on Vitamin K1

Vitamin K is relatively heat stable and doesn't get lost during cooking. In fact, cooking green leafy vegetables such as fresh chard and perilla leaf can actually increase their vitamin K concentrations. This is because plants store vitamin K in the chloroplast, and the cooking process breaks down the plant cell wall, which helps in the release of Vitamin K, resulting in a higher concentration of vitamin K in cooked leafy vegetables compared to raw vegetables.

Effect of Exposure to Light on Vitamin K1

While Vitamin K1 (phylloquinone) is unaffected by heat, it is highly sensitive to light and alkaline conditions. It is easily degraded by exposure to light and atmospheric oxygen and can be completely decomposed by alkalis. To keep your vitamin K-rich foods fresh and healthy, it's best to store them in dark-colored bottles to protect them from light.

It is recommended to avoid applying vitamin K to the skin, such as the face and hands, due to its instability in light. Without proper skin protection, exposure to light can cause vitamin K to cause photodegradation and phototoxicity in the skin. This is why the use of Vitamin K in cosmetic products is limited.

2.

IMPORTANCE OF VITAMIN K

FUNCTIONS OF VITAMIN K IN THE BODY

Role in Coagulation

The most important role of vitamin K in the body is its involvement in the blood clotting process. Vitamin K is required for the synthesis of proteins that are involved in blood clotting, such as prothrombin (clotting factor II) and clotting factors VII, IX, and X. Vitamin K acts as a coenzyme, enhancing the action of an enzyme required for the synthesis of these proteins. To form a clot, prothrombin in blood plasma is converted into thrombin by prothrombinase. Thrombin then converts fibrinogen into fibrin, which, together with platelets, creates a blood clot. This process is known as coagulation.

Have you ever noticed a dark brown hard coating on your wound 3-4 days after injury? This is known as blood clotting, a natural process that helps prevent excessive bleeding when you get hurt. Without blood clots, even a simple cut can increase your risk of bleeding to death. Blood clots also play a crucial role in reducing blood loss in situations such as trauma and cardiothoracic surgery. However, Blood clots can be beneficial or harmful, depending on the injury site. For instance, blood clotting at the outer surface of the body aids in stopping blood loss through the cut. But if a blood clot forms inside the body in blood vessels, it can be fatal since they do not dissolve naturally and require proper treatment.

Blood clotting can lead to life-threatening conditions like heart attacks and strokes when it occurs inside blood vessels and obstructs blood flow to vital organs. To prevent this, blood-thinning medications work by blocking the activity of vitamin K and stopping the formation of clots.

Role in Bone Metabolism

The process of bone metabolism involves a continuous cycle of bone growth and resorption. In order to preserve its strength and structure, bone requires constant remodeling. During this process, calcium is released from the bones into the bloodstream to meet other metabolic needs. This allows the bone to alter shape and size. The remodeling process persists throughout the lifetime, with bone reaching its peak mass and dominance by the early 20s. As a result of this continual process, the majority of the skeleton is replaced approximately every decade.

During the remodeling of bones, two types of cells are involved: osteoblasts, which form new bone, and osteoclasts, which break down old bone. As long as the process of bone formation (absorption) is greater than that of bone breakdown (resorption), the healthy bone structure is maintained.

Vitamin K is crucial for bone metabolism as it facilitates the gamma-carboxylation (activation) of several vitamin K-dependent proteins involved in bone health, such as osteocalcin, matrix Gla protein, and protein S. If these proteins are not carboxylated, they remain inactive and cannot contribute to the remodeling process. Additionally, vitamin K regulates the genetic transcription of osteoblastic markers and controls bone reabsorption.

Calcium is a crucial mineral for bone metabolism, and Vitamin K can have a positive impact on its balance. Osteocalcin, a protein, is responsible for transporting calcium from the bloodstream and binding it to the bone matrix, which ultimately increases bone strength and reduces the risk of fractures. However, osteocalcin is initially inactive, and its activation is necessary for it to be able to bind with calcium. For osteocalcin to attract calcium, gamma-carboxylation is essential, allowing it to bind with calcium and concentrate in the bone. Vitamin K plays an important role in activating osteocalcin and preventing the accumulation of calcium on blood vessel walls. This ensures that calcium is deposited in bones rather than in the walls of blood vessels.

Vitamin K insufficiency results in an increase in the concentration of undercarboxylated osteocalcin (ucOC) in blood circulation. As a result, calcium remains in blood circulation and doesn't get concentrated in bone, which results in hip fracture, especially in older people due to bone loss. This is why The Institute of Medicine has increased the dietary reference intakes of vitamin K by approximately 50% from previous recommendations to 90 mcg per day for females and 120 mcg per day for males.

Although vitamin K from natural sources has positive effects on bone health, studies so far have not found any remarkable improvement in bone mineral density with supplements of vitamin K1 and vitamin K2. Therefore, taking vitamin K supplements for bones is not recommended, and any such claims are neither scientifically supported nor authorized by official bodies. To improve bone health, it is recommended to increase the consumption of vitamin K1 and K2-rich foods.

Role in Heart Health

Calcification refers to the accumulation of calcium in body tissues. While calcium is necessary for bone formation, it can also have negative effects. When calcium is deposited abnormally on the walls of blood vessels, it can cause them to become hardened and potentially lead to fatal consequences.

Vitamin K, particularly vitamin K2, plays a crucial role in maintaining a healthy heart. It prevents calcium from depositing on the walls of blood vessels, thereby inhibiting arterial calcification and stiffening. Vitamin K activates a protein called matrix GLA protein (MGP), which is produced by the cells of vascular smooth muscles and acts as a central calcification inhibitor. By preventing the accumulation of calcium salts, vitamin K helps keep the heart healthy.

To get maximum health benefits, it is recommended to consume vitamin K with vitamin D. Consuming vitamin K with vitamin D is more effective for cardiovascular and bone health compared to consuming either alone. This is because these two vitamins work together synergistically. Vitamin D aids in the production of vitamin K-dependent protein, which is essential for proper carboxylation. Additionally, Vitamin D increases calcium absorption in the body and strengthens the bones.

Maintaining sufficient calcium levels in your blood is crucial for many bodily functions. If you don't consume enough calcium, vitamin D will extract calcium from your bones to maintain adequate levels in your blood. This can lead to bone loss and osteoporosis over time. To ensure that calcium is properly deposited in your bones rather than elsewhere in your body, it's important to consume vitamin D through natural sources with vitamin K. Vitamin K helps regulate calcium in your body by activating osteocalcin, which promotes calcium accumulation in your bones, as well as activating matrix GLA protein (MGP), which prevents calcium from depositing in soft tissues like blood vessels.

Role in Cancer Protection

Cancer is the second leading cause of mortality worldwide after heart disease. Many research studies have proved that vitamin K has antitumor effects. High intake of vitamin K is directly linked with lower cancer risks.

All types of vitamin K (vitamin K1, vitamin K2, and vitamin K3) can positively suppress cancer growth and differentiation. Vitamin K inhibits several cancer cell lines by inducing apoptosis and cell cycle arrest of cancer cells at different levels. The cell cycle of cancer cells represents a survival mechanism that allows the tumor cell to repair its damaged DNA. Thus, before DNA repair is complete, vitamin K abolishes the cell cycle checkpoints that cause an apoptosis cascade, leading to cancer cell death.

Out of the three types of vitamin K, vitamin K3 is the most potent but also highly toxic, making it unsuitable for cancer treatment. On the other hand, vitamin K2 has a milder effect than K3 but without any side effects, while vitamin K1 has the least function. Therefore, vitamin K2 is a potential chemotherapeutic candidate for cancer treatment. Vitamin K2 has been found to have anticancer effects against various types of cancer, such as, lung cancer, liver cancer, bile duct cancer, leukemia, pancreatic cancer, ovarian cancer, and colorectal cancer.

When used alone, Vitamin K2 has shown positive results in cancer treatment. However, its effects become even stronger when combined with other chemotherapy drugs.

One such drug is Retinoids, which can be used in cancer treatment. The combination of Vitamin K2 and Retinoids has been found to produce synergistic effects. Retinoids work by suppressing the growth of cancer cells, while Vitamin K2 enhances their effectiveness. This combination has also been shown to decrease the recurrence rate of hepatocellular carcinoma (HCC), the most common type of liver cancer.

Another micronutrient, vitamin D3, can reduce the growth of cancer cells by inhibiting cell proliferation and stimulating cell differentiation. However, a potential side effect of vitamin D3 is that it can increase the concentration of calcium in your blood, leading to calcium buildup in your vascular system and increasing the risk of blood clots and stroke. To counteract this, vitamin K2 can regulate calcium deposition and ensure it gets deposited in bone tissue rather than building up in the vascular system. When combined with vitamin D3, vitamin K2 can reduce the risk of calcium buildup and vascular calcification. Additionally, this combination can enhance the induction of cellular differentiation in cancer cells through their synergistic effect.

Health Benefits of Eating Vitamin K

Healing a Wound

The consumption of vitamin K, particularly vitamin K1, may enhance the rate of wound healing. In total, thirteen proteins are required for blood clotting, with vitamin K contributing to four of them. By promoting the formation of blood clots, vitamin K prevents excessive bleeding from wounds and speeds up the recovery process.

Prevent Fracture Incidence

Studies have shown that vitamin K deficiency can increase the likelihood of fractures. This is because vitamin K plays a crucial role in regulating calcium deposition and ensuring that it is properly deposited in bones rather than circulating in the blood. This helps to maintain bone mineral density and prevent fractures. It is especially important for individuals over 70, as they are more susceptible to bone loss and require higher vitamin K levels to reduce fracture incidents. Therefore, consuming enough vitamin K-rich foods is important to maintain strong and healthy bones.

Prevent Osteoporosis

Osteoporosis is a condition that makes your bones weak and easy to break, increasing the risk of fractures. This happens when old bone loss exceeds new bone formation, leading to lower bone mineral density and mass. As bone mass decreases, bones become more vulnerable to fractures. Vitamin K is an essential nutrient for bone health. It effectively reduces fracture rates in people with osteoporosis and increases bone mineral density. Vitamin K activates bone proteins and regulates calcium deposition in bones, which strengthens them. Adding vitamin K-rich foods, calcium, and vitamin D to your diet can reduce the risk of developing osteoporosis.

Improve Heart Health

Consuming adequate amounts of Vitamin K2 can effectively reduce the risk of vascular damage. Vitamin K2 activates matrix GLA protein (MGP), which prevents calcium deposition in blood vessel walls. This helps utilize calcium for other essential bodily functions, promoting the health and flexibility of arteries. Increasing your vitamin K intake may help lower the health risks associated with high calcium levels.

Prevent Kidney Stone Formation

Excessive calcium intake can result in the formation of kidney stones. Conversely, a deficiency in vitamin K can also increase your likelihood of developing kidney stones. By ensuring an adequate intake of vitamin K, calcium buildup in the kidneys can be prevented. Vitamin K plays a key role in regulating calcium levels in the body and activates matrix GLA protein (MGP), which prevents calcium accumulation in soft tissues, including the kidneys.

Boost Cognitive Health

Lower Vitamin K levels have been linked to cognitive dysfunction. Vitamin K is crucial for enhancing cognitive health as it has an anti-apoptotic effect, which means it helps prevent cell death. Research indicates that vitamin K intake can decrease the risk of Alzheimer's disease due to this effect. Additionally, it can reduce inflammation in the brain and spinal cord, improve mitochondrial function, and positively impact conditions like Parkinson's and Multiple Sclerosis. Vitamin K also acts as a co-factor in the synthesis of sphingolipids, which are essential components of brain cell membranes. These lipids play a vital role in regulating cell proliferation, differentiation, and survival.

Research indicates that the use of blood thinning medication can greatly reduce both visual memory and verbal fluency. For those taking medication that acts as a vitamin K antagonist, it is important to maintain a healthy intake of vitamin K through diet, as the use of such medication can result in cognitive decline.

Is there anything I should be aware of?

If you're taking blood-thinning medication, consuming sufficient amounts of vitamin K-rich foods is important. These medications work by inhibiting the activity of vitamin K, which can lead to lower-than-normal levels of this nutrient. Maintaining consistent vitamin K intake can help prevent other health issues that may arise from a deficiency.

INTERACTION

Vitamin K interactions with other drugs:

Anti-Coagulating Medications with Vitamin K

Excessive intake of vitamin K does not cause abnormal blood clotting. There is no known toxicity associated with the intake of either vitamin K1 or vitamin K2. However, if you are at a high risk of developing blood clots and are taking prescribed blood-thinning medications (anticoagulants) to prevent clot formation in organs such as the heart, kidney, lungs, and soft tissue, it is important to maintain a consistent and same amount of vitamin K intake through your diet.

Certain blood-thinning medications, such as warfarin, work by counteracting the effect of vitamin K, which can lead to a deficiency in vitamin K. As Vitamin K has blood clotting effects, it can interfere with the effectiveness of blood thinning medications. If you're taking anticoagulation drugs, sudden changes in your vitamin K intake can have serious consequences. Consuming too much vitamin K can cause blood clots while consuming too little can lead to excessive bleeding. It's recommended that people taking anticoagulants consume a sustained intake of vitamin K through food, meeting current dietary recommendations of 90-120 µg/day. However, it's important to consult your doctor and pharmacist before making any major changes to your vitamin K intake.

Antibiotics and Vitamin K

Antibiotics have two modes of action, either by killing bacteria or by halting their growth. In the process of eliminating harmful bacteria, antibiotics may also eliminate good bacteria that produce vitamin K in the gut. This may result in a decrease in overall vitamin K levels. Some types of antibiotics, such as cephalosporin antibiotics (cefoperazone), are more likely to cause this effect because they not only kill vitamin K-producing bacteria but also hinder the absorption of vitamin K in the body. Vitamin K supplements are often prescribed with cephalosporin antibiotics when these antibiotics are prescribed for more than ten days. However, if the antibiotics are only used for short periods, supplements are not typically necessary.

Anti-Seizure Medications and Vitamin K

Phenytoin is a commonly used anticonvulsant drug to manage various types of seizures. However, it can impede the body's ability to utilize vitamin K by triggering vitamin K metabolism. This may lead to a vitamin K deficiency, which can result in bone loss, osteoporosis, and bleeding incidents. If taken during pregnancy, anticonvulsants like phenytoin may also cause vitamin K deficiency in newborns. Studies have shown that babies born to mothers who took anticonvulsant drugs during pregnancy had lower vitamin K levels in their blood, putting them at risk of bleeding.

Weight-Loss Medications and Vitamin K

Weight-loss drug, orlistat, is a lipase inhibitor that is used in the management of obesity. This drug works by inhibiting gastric and pancreatic lipases, which are responsible for digesting dietary fat. As a result, orlistat decreases the absorption of dietary fat in the body. However, orlistat can also lower the absorption of fat-soluble vitamins, including vitamin K. To prevent any issues, it is common for doctors to prescribe a multivitamin supplement that contains vitamin K with orlistat. If you are taking blood thinners along with orlistat, it may affect your vitamin K status. It is recommended to consult with your doctor and pharmacist to address any potential risk of Vitamin K deficiency.

Olestra and Vitamin K

Olestra is a fat substitute that has been approved by the FDA for use in savory snacks. The Olestra molecule is created from soybean or cottonseed oil and is much larger than regular fat molecules. This makes it impossible for the body to digest and absorb it, resulting in it passing through the body undigested without adding any trans-fat, cholesterol, and calories to your body. FDA has approved its use in potato chips, corn chips, tortillas, crackers, and ready-to-eat popcorn!

Consuming foods containing olestra can lower the absorption of fat-soluble vitamins, including vitamin K. To address this issue, the Food and Drug Administration now requires that food products containing olestra have vitamin K and other fat-soluble vitamins (A, D, and E) added to them. This is to compensate for any potential reduction in absorption caused by olestra's action.

Cholesterol-Lowering Drugs and Vitamin K

Medications that lower cholesterol, such as bile acid sequestrants, work by preventing the absorption of bile acids from the stomach into the bloodstream, which helps lower LDL cholesterol in the body. However, these medications can also decrease the absorption of fat-soluble vitamins like vitamin K, which could cause a deficiency. Examples of bile acid sequestrants include cholestyramine, colesevelam, and colestipol. If you take these medications for a prolonged period, it is important to have your vitamin K levels checked.

3.

10 RICHEST FOOD SOURCES OF VITAMIN K

Here are the top 10 foods that are high in Vitamin K:

1. Mustard Green

Mustard greens are among the richest sources of vitamin K. Cooked mustard greens have more vitamin K than raw ones. 100 gm of cooked mustard greens can provide you with 564% of your daily vitamin K requirement. These greens are incredibly beneficial for your health. They are low in calories, with about 92% water, and are packed with essential nutrients such as vitamins A, C, and E, calcium, and powerful phytonutrients. Consuming mustard greens regularly can improve your eye health, bone health, and brain functions and even reduce your risk of chronic diseases such as autoimmune diseases and heart diseases. Additionally, these greens act as detoxifying agents that help purify your blood and promote healthy skin.

2. Spinach

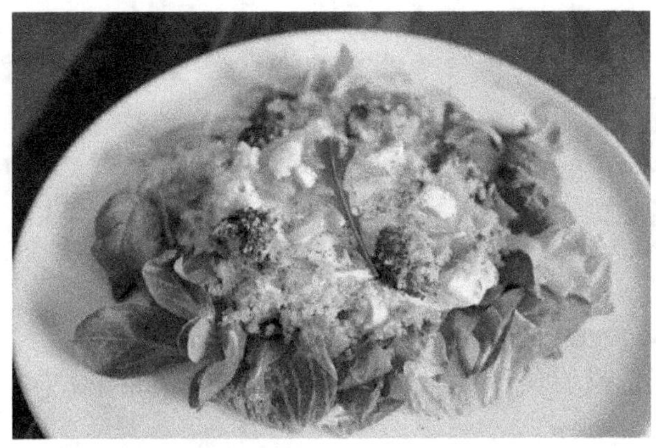

Spinach is packed with vitamins and minerals. This superfood is high in vitamins K, A, and C and in minerals such as calcium, iron, potassium, and manganese. Half a cup of cooked spinach gives you an incredible 370% of your daily vitamin K requirement, three times the amount you need in a day. Additionally, spinach's anti-inflammatory and antioxidant properties can help protect you from various chronic diseases. Adding spinach to your diet ensures your body's functions run smoothly, and you feel energized and refreshed all day.

Spinach is packed with essential nutrients that are hard to ignore, even if you aren't fond of its distinctive flavor. It's time to get creative and find some exciting ways to incorporate spinach into your meals. To make it more palatable, add low-fat cream, butter, tomatoes, or lime juice while cooking spinach. Adding lime juice or tomatoes can enhance the absorption of iron while incorporating healthy fats can improve the absorption of fat-soluble vitamins A, E, and K.

Other dark leafy vegetables that are excellent sources of vitamin K are

Cooked collards: Half cup contains 442% of the daily value.

Cooked turnip greens: Half a cup contains 355% of the daily value.

Raw Kale: One cup contains 94% of the daily value.

Lettuce: 100 grams contain 97% of daily value.

3. Broccoli

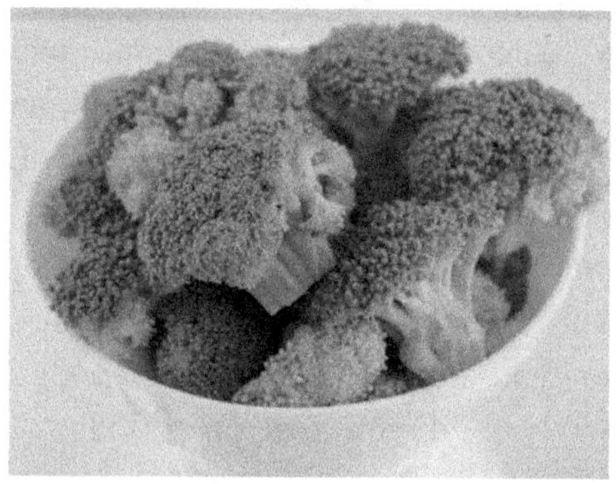

Broccoli is a cruciferous vegetable that is packed with vitamin K and vitamin C. Half a cup of cooked broccoli gives you 92% of your daily recommended vitamin K. For maximum vitamin K intake, cook broccoli with oils like mustard, canola, or soybean oil, which are naturally rich in this nutrient. Not only does broccoli help build strong bones due to its high vitamin K and moderate calcium content, but it also contains sulforaphane, which can help prevent osteoporosis. Additionally, pregnant women should eat plenty of broccoli as it is an excellent source of folate, a crucial nutrient for the proper development of the baby's brain and spinal cord. Other cruciferous vegetables like cauliflower, cabbage, or Brussels sprouts are also rich in Vitamin **K.**

4. Okra/ Lady' Fingers

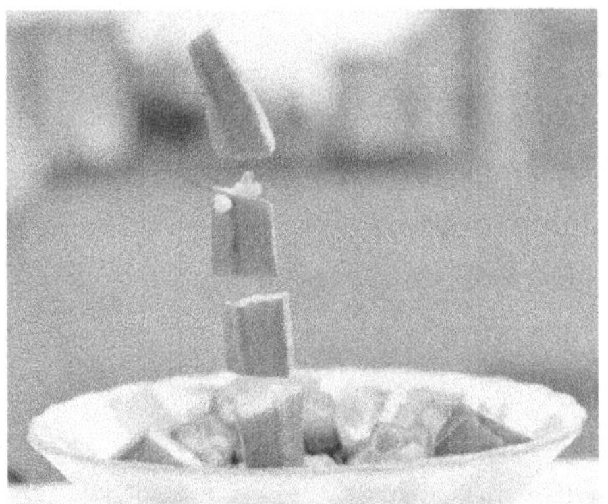

Do you know that okra, commonly known as lady's fingers, is actually a fruit and not a vegetable? It's packed with essential nutrients such as vitamin K, vitamin C, and dietary fiber. One cup of raw okra contains 26% of the daily requirement of vitamin K and is low in calories while providing significant amounts of vitamin B1, B9, magnesium, and calcium. Okra is rich in potent antioxidants, such as polyphenols, which help combat free radicals and prevent heart problems and stroke. It also contains lectin, a type of protein that has anticancer properties and can inhibit cancer cell growth.

For people with diabetes, okra is a great choice due to its high dietary fiber content. Research has found that the viscous soluble dietary fiber in okra can help reduce the absorption of sugar in the intestine, resulting in a gradual release of sugar into the bloodstream preventing a sudden rise in blood sugar levels. However, if you are taking diabetes medication, such as metformin, it's important to limit your consumption of okra as it can decrease the absorption of the medication, making it less effective in controlling blood sugar levels. You should consult with your doctor before adding okra to your diet.

5. Soybean

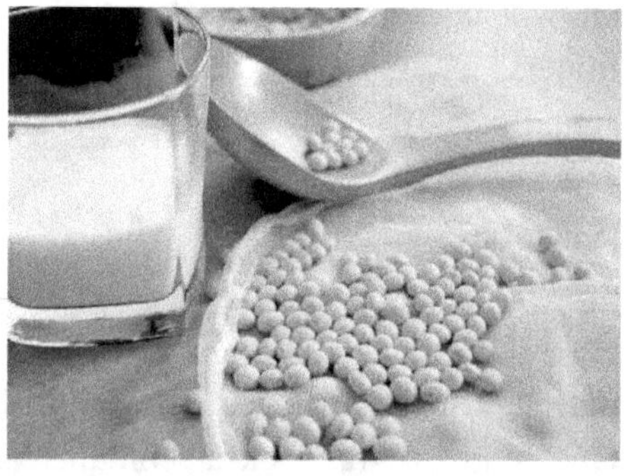

Soybeans are highly nutritious. They are rich in Vitamin K, Vitamin B, iron, fiber, manganese, and phosphorus. Half a cup of cooked soybeans can fulfill 36% of your daily vitamin K requirement, and one tablespoon of soybean oil contains 21% of the daily value of vitamin K. Not only that, but they also contain all nine essential amino acids that your body needs for proper function, making them an excellent source of complete protein. However, to ensure optimal digestion, it's important to soak the soybeans overnight or for at least 8-10 hours before cooking them well in enough water. This is because soybeans contain trypsin inhibitors that can prevent protein digestion and limit the health benefits of the soybeans. Trypsin is an enzyme needed to break down protein, making it easier for the body to absorb. Soaking and cooking the beans properly destroys these inhibitors, allowing better digestion and nutrient absorption.

6. Green Peas

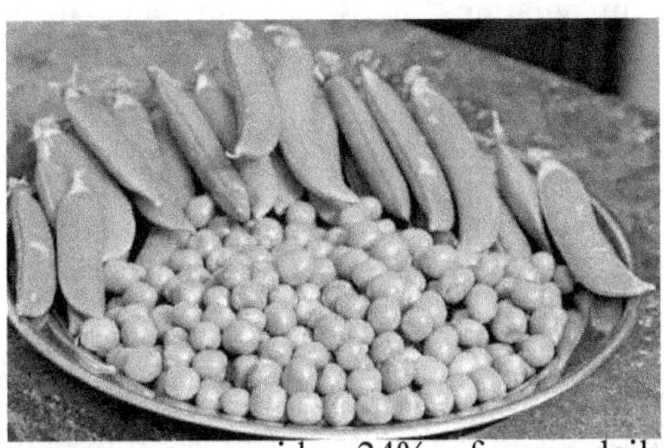

Green peas are an excellent source of various vitamins and minerals. 100 grams of raw green peas provides 24% of your daily recommended intake of vitamin K. These peas also contain decent amounts of vitamins A, B1, B9, and C, as well as essential minerals like manganese, zinc, and iron. Furthermore, they're rich in fiber and protein, which can help you feel full for longer and potentially aid in weight loss. However, it's important to cook green peas thoroughly because raw ones contain antinutrients like lectin, which can cause bloating and digestive issues when consumed in large quantities, and phytic acid, which can reduce the absorption of vital minerals like iron, zinc, and calcium. Cooking green peas reduces the levels of lectin and phytic acid.

7. Sprouted Mung Beans

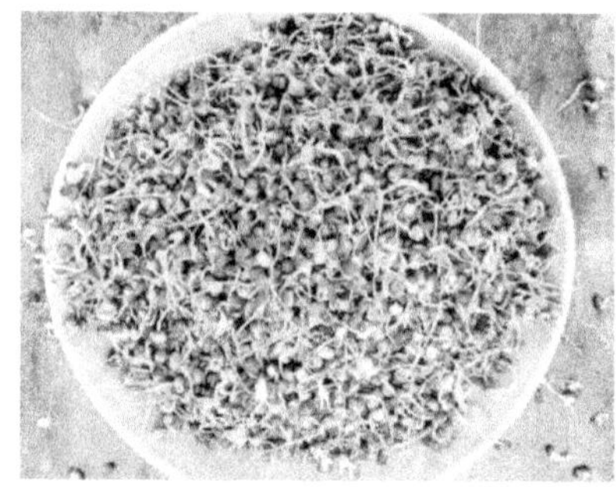

Sprouted mung beans are a popular choice as compared to other sprouts. When mung beans are sprouted, their nutritional value increases by up to 100%. Sprouted mung beans are rich in vitamins K, C, folate, and iron. Furthermore, sprouted mung beans have more antioxidants and amino acids. A 100-gram serving of raw sprouted mung beans contains 27% of the recommended daily value of vitamin K. It is recommended to sprout mung beans at home instead of buying them from a store, as the latter may be contaminated with bacteria. If you do use store-bought sprouts, it is important to cook them well, as this may reduce the nutritional value, but effectively kill any potential bacteria. For maximum health benefits, it is recommended that you sprout mung beans at home, as this process is simple and does not require specific environmental conditions.

Some other vegetables that can provide you with a good amount of vitamin K include cooked French beans, which contain 25% of the daily value in half a cup, and pumpkin, which has 17% of the daily value in half a cup.

8. Carrot Juice

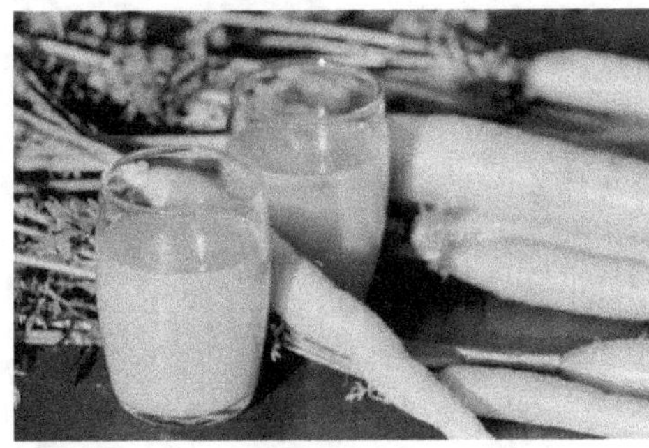

Carrots aren't just a great source of vitamin A, but they're also rich in vitamin K. Drinking just ¾ cup of carrot juice can fulfill 23% of your daily vitamin K requirement. Not only do carrots keep your eyes healthy, but they also provide cardiovascular protection. The high content of different carotenoids in carrots has potent antioxidant effects that can neutralize free radicals, reduce the risk of chronic diseases, and protect against several types of cancer, including stomach, colon, and prostate cancers. If you want to maximize the health benefits of carrots, consider choosing red ones because they contain more lycopene, a powerful antioxidant that can improve heart health, protect your skin from sun damage, improve fertility in young men, and lower the risk of bone, lung, and prostate cancers.

9. Kiwi

Not just an apple consuming a kiwi daily may also decrease the frequency of doctor

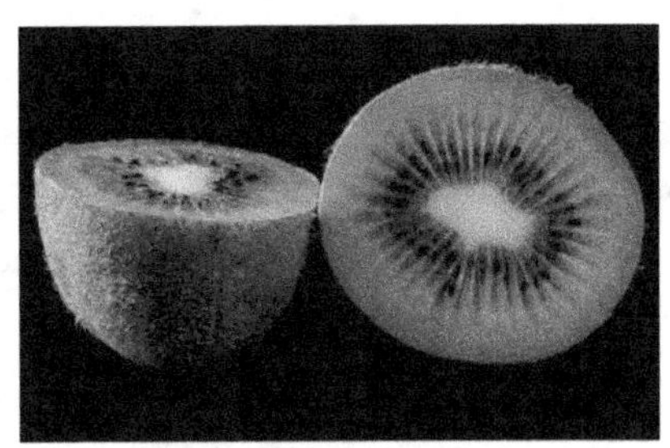

visits. Kiwis are an excellent source of vitamin C and provide a moderate amount of vitamins K and E. A single medium-sized kiwi contains 23% of the recommended daily intake of vitamin K. Kiwis are high in fiber, promoting healthy digestion. Studies have shown that consuming kiwis may help with sleep onset, duration, and efficiency for individuals with sleep disturbances. Additionally, kiwis can improve iron absorption in the body and maintain healthy blood cells. Eating a kiwi daily can provide sustained energy throughout the day.

10. Pomegranate

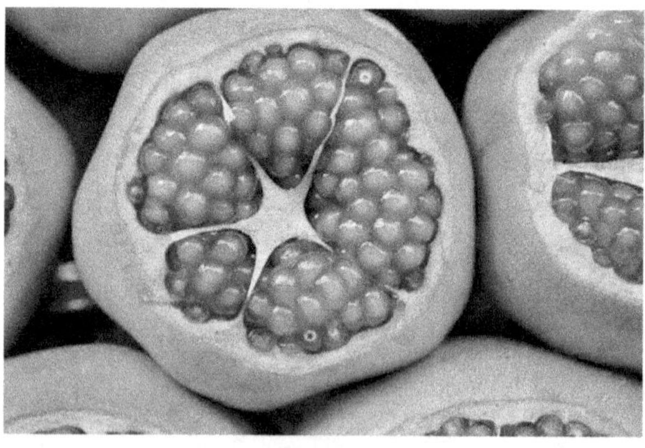

Pomegranates are a highly nutritious fruit. Not only are the arils packed with nutrients, but the peel is equally nutritious. One large pomegranate can provide 45% of your daily recommended intake of vitamin K. Pomegranates also contain polyphenols, a type of phytochemicals that plants produce to protect themselves against fungi, bacteria, and virus infections. When you eat foods rich in phytochemicals, like pomegranates, they act as antioxidants in your body and have anti-inflammatory effects. The polyphenols in pomegranates help prevent the formation of free radicals, reduce oxidative damage to cells, and decrease inflammation in the body. This can be helpful in protecting against diseases like arthritis, heart disease, and Alzheimer's disease. Pomegranate peel has a high phenolic content and is used in making dietary supplements.

Vitamin K2

Some natural sources of Vitamin K2 (MK-4) include cheddar cheese, mozzarella cheese, milk, yogurt, and miso. While they may not be the most significant sources of vitamin K, it is still important to include them in your diet to meet your body's vitamin K requirements.

UNIT 3

VITAMIN COMBINATIONS - DOS AND DON'TS

When taking vitamins, it's important to consider how different combinations may affect the body. For vitamins to produce their intended effects, they must be adequately absorbed in the body. Combining certain vitamins with other vitamins, medications, or minerals can either enhance or hinder their absorption rates. Some vitamin combinations may have a synergistic effect, increasing the absorption of other vitamins and providing better health benefits than if taken alone. However, other combinations may compete for absorption in the body, nullifying their effects and potentially causing toxicity.

Let's take a look at the beneficial and dangerous combination of vitamins that can affect your health in many ways.

Chapter 1

POTENTIALLY DANGEROUS VITAMIN COMBINATIONS YOU SHOULD AVOID

VITAMIN E + VITAMIN K

Vitamin K is important for maintaining bone health, promoting wound healing, and aiding blood clotting. However, when taken with vitamin E, the effects of Vitamin K can be reduced. Vitamin E has blood thinning effects and also increases the metabolism of Vitamin K in the liver, which leads to increased excretion of all forms of vitamin K. While consuming vitamin K-rich foods like spinach and kale with vitamin E-rich foods like nuts or vegetable oil in moderation may not have adverse effects, high intake of vitamin E-rich foods or taking Vitamin E supplements alongside Vitamin K supplements can diminish the benefits of Vitamin K in the body.

VITAMIN A + VITAMIN K

Consuming excessive amounts of Vitamin A can hinder Vitamin K absorption in the body, which is necessary for effective blood clotting. However, consuming vitamin A-rich foods in moderation is unlikely to have a significant impact on Vitamin K absorption, but taking high doses of Vitamin A supplements may significantly decrease the effectiveness of vitamin K.

HIGH DOSE OF VITAMIN D + MAGNESIUM

It's important to take the right amounts of Vitamin D and magnesium, even though they are an ideal combination. Taking too many Vitamin D supplements can be harmful, as it can lead to toxic levels of Vitamin D in the blood. This can result in a depletion of magnesium. However, when you get your Vitamin D from food sources or sunlight, it's less likely to reach those toxic levels. If you take high doses of Vitamin D for an extended period, it can lead to calcium build-up in the blood, which is known as hypercalcemia. This can potentially increase magnesium excretion through urine, leading to magnesium volume depletion in the body.

VITAMIN E AND A + BLOOD THINNERS

If you are taking an anticoagulant or blood-thinning medication, such as warfarin, limiting your consumption of foods rich in Vitamin E and Vitamin A is important. This is because taking Vitamin E or A with blood-thinning medication may increase the risk of bleeding events, which can be particularly dangerous if you are also taking Vitamin E or A supplements. However, some studies suggest that Vitamin E supplements can be safely taken by individuals who require chronic warfarin therapy. It is recommended to maintain a 2-hour gap between taking warfarin and Vitamin E or A supplements. Alternatively, you should consult your doctor and pharmacist regarding your supplement and food consumption while taking blood-thinning medication.

VITAMIN K + BLOOD THINNERS

Vitamin K interferes with the way anticoagulants like warfarin work. Vitamin K is a coagulant, which means it helps your blood clot, while warfarin is designed to prevent blood clots. Eating foods rich in Vitamin K can make your medication less effective, so limiting your consumption of these foods while on blood thinning drug therapy is important. Additionally, it's important to keep your Vitamin K intake consistent to ensure the effectiveness of your therapy. Avoid eating vitamin K-rich foods within 2 hours of taking your medication. It is recommended to seek advice from your doctor and pharmacist before altering your diet or beginning any medication or vitamin supplements.

FAT-SOLUBLE VITAMINS + WATER-SOLUBLE VITAMINS

In order to receive the health benefits of vitamins, they must be properly absorbed. It's not recommended to take fat-soluble vitamins (A, D, E, and K) with water-soluble vitamins (B complex and C) because they are absorbed differently in the body. Combining them may reduce the health benefits you receive from each. Water-soluble vitamins are well absorbed on an empty stomach, while fat-soluble vitamins require the presence of fat in the body to be adequately absorbed. To maximize the benefits of each type of vitamin, consume B and C-rich foods in the morning and foods rich in A, D, E, and K in the evening. If you take vitamin supplements, take B and C on an empty stomach and take fat-soluble vitamins in the evening after a meal.

Chapter 2

VITAMIN COMBINATIONS FOR SYNERGISTIC HEALTH BENEFITS

VITAMIN D + CALCIUM

You may have noticed that calcium supplements usually come in combination with vitamin D. This is because both nutrients are crucial for maintaining strong and healthy bones. Vitamin D plays a critical role in calcium absorption, increasing its absorption by two times. If your body lacks Vitamin D, it cannot efficiently absorb calcium. This results in an insufficient amount of calcium for your body's needs. Consequently, your body may extract calcium from your bones to meet its other needs, which can weaken your bones, hinder new bone growth, and increase the risk of fractures.

The relationship between vitamin D and calcium is interconnected. It's not just that vitamin D impacts the availability of calcium in the body, but calcium also affects the availability of vitamin D. Insufficient calcium intake elevates the likelihood of vitamin D deficiency. Conversely, consuming high levels of calcium guarantees that vitamin D remains available in the body for a more extended period.

To receive maximum health benefits, spend 10 to 30 minutes in the sun in the morning and follow up with a glass of milk or other calcium-rich foods like yogurt, soybeans, spinach, kale, figs, papaya, and oranges.

VITAMIN D + MAGNESIUM

Optimum intake of magnesium helps to overcome vitamin D deficiency. Studies show that increasing magnesium consumption in individuals with vitamin D deficiency can boost their vitamin D levels. Magnesium is crucial for vitamin D synthesis, activation, regulation, and transportation. Vitamin D remains inactive until it is converted by enzymes in the liver and kidney into its active form. For these enzymes to work effectively, they require magnesium. Without it, the enzymes cannot efficiently convert inactive vitamin D into its active form, and you miss out on its health benefits. In return, Vitamin D promotes magnesium absorption in the body, particularly in those with low magnesium levels.

Combining magnesium and vitamin D is crucial for optimal health as they work together to improve various functions within the body. This powerful duo strengthens the immune system, promotes healthy bone growth, and alleviates muscle spasms. Also, this life-saving combination reduces the risk of insulin resistance, type 2 diabetes, and hypertension by many folds. Magnesium-rich foods that you can combine with vitamin D are a handful of pumpkin seeds, chia seeds, cashews, peanuts, spinach, kale, brown rice, and yogurt.

VITAMIN K2 + VITAMIN D

To boost your bone health and cardiovascular health, it is recommended to consume both vitamin K and vitamin D together. These fat-soluble vitamins play an important role in calcium metabolism. When taken together, they are more effective in increasing bone density and reducing the risk of fractures compared to when taken alone.   Vitamin D helps increase the concentration of bone proteins such as osteocalcin and Gla protein (BGP), which are responsible for bone formation. However, these proteins remain inactive and require vitamin K to be converted into their active form. Osteocalcin then binds to calcium and helps transport it from the blood to the bones. Without enough vitamin K and vitamin D, calcium may not be absorbed into the bone and instead get deposited in the arteries, affecting bone and cardiovascular health. Vitamin K reduces calcium excretion through urine, while vitamin D increases intestinal calcium absorption and prevents hypocalcemia. Vitamin K2 - MK-4 is effective for bone health, while MK-7 is beneficial for cardiovascular health.

Vitamin D deficiency, along with vitamin K deficiency, increases your risk of hypertension and diabetes. Having both vitamins together can help keep the blood pressure normal. Furthermore, vitamins D and K can improve insulin secretion and beta-cell proliferation in the pancreas, and provide protection against cardiovascular diseases.

For optimal results, it is advisable to obtain vitamins from diet rather than relying on dietary supplements. Overconsumption of vitamin D supplements may even increase the risk of cardiovascular diseases. This is due to the fact that excessive vitamin D intake can cause an increase in vitamin D-dependent proteins, which require vitamin K to activate. Without sufficient vitamin K, these proteins cannot be activated. Therefore, they cannot stimulate bone mineralization or inhibit soft tissue calcification. This can ultimately lead to bone fractures and cardiovascular diseases. If you are taking blood thinners like warfarin (a vitamin K antagonist) while also taking vitamin D supplements, it is crucial to consult your doctor regarding the appropriate dosage of your vitamin D supplements. To get the maximum health benefits, add more vegetables and fermented dairy into your diet for bone and cardiovascular health.

VITAMIN E + OMEGA-3 FATS

Reducing inflammation in the body is important to prevent chronic disorders such as hypertension, type 2 diabetes, kidney disease, and cardiovascular disease. Omega-3 fatty acids help in reducing inflammation.

Vitamin E has potent antioxidant effects, which protect cells from damage caused by free radicals and limit their harmful effects. Vitamin E also provides protection against cancer and cardiovascular diseases while enhancing the immune system.

Omega-3 fatty acids, such as alpha-linolenic acid (ALA), eicosapentaenoic acid (EPA), and docosahexaenoic acid (DHA), are polyunsaturated (PUFA) and are prone to oxidation in the gut. Omega-3-rich foods like flaxseeds, chia seeds, and canola oil can even be oxidized during processing and storage, which reduces their stability and health benefits. Oxidized Omega-3 fatty acids cause oxidative stress and have deteriorating effects on the body. However, combining antioxidants like vitamin E with Omega 3 can prevent its oxidation and increase its stability in the gut.

For maximum health benefits, it's recommended to consume foods that are high in vitamin E, like sunflower seeds, almonds, peanuts, pumpkin, spinach, and mangoes, with omega-3 fats-rich foods, such as flaxseeds, chia seeds, walnuts, and kidney beans.

VITAMIN D + OMEGA-3 FATS

Recent research has shown that the combination of vitamin D and omega-3 fats can provide greater protection against heart attacks, strokes, and cancer, although its effectiveness for preventing these diseases in those who already have them or are at higher risk is mixed. Studies indicate that incorporating vitamin D3 and omega-3 fatty acid-rich foods into your diet, along with light exercise, can lower the risk of cancer in the general population. This combination is particularly effective for physically active individuals over the age of 70.

In addition, the combination of omega-3 fatty acids and vitamin D has a synergic impact on mental health and can enhance cognitive function by affecting the serotonin system. Serotonin is a neurotransmitter that contributes to optimism, happiness, and contentment. If your body is deficient in vitamin D and omega-3 fatty acids, it can lead to low serotonin levels, which increases the likelihood of developing psychiatric conditions such as depression, mood swings, dementia, autism, bipolar disorder, and schizophrenia. By working in conjunction with vitamin D, omega fats like docosahexaenoic acid (DHA) and eicosapentaenoic acid (EPA) help regulate serotonin levels in the brain. Vitamin D is involved in serotonin synthesis, EPA increases serotonin release, and DHA influences serotonin receptor action. Together, these factors improve serotonin levels in the body, promoting overall happiness and reducing the risk of psychiatric disorders.

Incorporate omega-3-rich foods like seaweed, flaxseed, chia seeds, walnuts, and soybean oil into your diet, and pair them with vitamin D-rich foods such as milk and milk products. Additionally, make sure to get plenty of early morning sunlight.

VITAMIN K + CALCIUM

Bone mineral density (BMD) indicates the amount of calcium and other minerals in your bones. When you don't get enough calcium, your BMD can decrease and increase your risk of bone fractures. Calcium is not only important for bones but also for the proper function of muscles and nerves. It acts as factor IV and plays a critical role in blood clotting. However, too much calcium in the body (often caused by high doses of calcium supplements) can be harmful and increase your risk of heart disease. Excess calcium can accumulate in the walls of your blood vessels, blocking the smooth blood flow and leading to heart attacks and strokes.

The amount of vitamin K in the body has a direct impact on calcium levels. If you are low in vitamin K, it can negatively affect your bone metabolism and lead to osteoporosis and fractures. Even with enough calcium in the body, low vitamin K levels can prevent proper utilization of calcium. This can cause calcium deposits in blood vessels instead of bones, which increases the risk of weak bones and heart disease. A combination of calcium and vitamin K is essential for high bone mineral density (BMR) and better heart health. Eating calcium-rich foods like kale and okra, along with vitamin K-rich foods like cheese and fermented foods like natto, can help promote stronger bones and a healthier heart.

VITAMIN E + VITAMIN C

Both vitamin E and vitamin C have antioxidant properties, but they differ in solubility. Vitamin C is a water-soluble antioxidant, while vitamin E is a lipid-soluble antioxidant. When combined, these two vitamins can boost immunity, reduce the risk of developing chronic diseases, and protect against exercise-induced damage.

Vitamin E is a potent antioxidant. However, when combined with Vitamin C, it becomes even more effective. Vitamin E's main role is to act as a lipid antioxidant, which helps protect the polyunsaturated fatty acids (PUFAs) found in the membrane from lipid peroxidation. When free radicals attack these PUFAs, it can lead to cell damage. Vitamin E can prevent this by binding with free radicals and rendering them ineffective. However, this process also causes Vitamin E to change into a form that can no longer bind with other free radicals. Luckily, Vitamin C can solve this problem.

Vitamin C helps recycle vitamin E. Vitamin C enhances vitamin E's antioxidant activity, making it more efficient. After vitamin E binds with free radicals and becomes oxidized, vitamin C steps in and reduces it back to its original form of tocopherol. With vitamin E restored, it can bind with free radicals again, rendering them ineffective. Together, vitamin C and vitamin E form an antioxidant network that protects against chronic diseases by safeguarding lipids, proteins, and DNA against free radical damage.

Studies indicate that consuming foods that are rich in vitamins E and C can lower the risk of reduced lung function or asthma, particularly in people who are at an increased risk of developing these conditions, such as smokers. However, taking supplements of both vitamins did not yield the same results. The combination of vitamins E and C supplements has produced mixed results, and further studies are needed to draw a definitive conclusion.

For maximum health benefits, incorporate vitamin C-rich foods like citrus fruits, strawberries, and tomatoes, as well as vitamin E foods such as almonds, sunflower oil, pumpkin, and red bell peppers into your diet. However, it is not advisable to consume water-soluble vitamins like vitamin C with fat-soluble vitamins. Therefore, it is recommended to maintain a gap of 2-3 hours between the consumption of both types of vitamins.

VITAMIN A + IRON

A lack of Vitamin A can have an impact on iron metabolism, which can lead to anemia. Although Vitamin A deficiency does not decrease iron absorption, it can reduce the synthesis of hemoglobin. To combat anemia, it is recommended to consume foods that are high in both iron and vitamin A. Studies have shown that combining vitamin A with iron is more effective in increasing hemoglobin levels than consuming iron alone.

This is because Vitamin A enhances iron utilization in the body.

Let's understand the science behind it:

Seeds, legumes, and grains like wheat, rice, and corn (yes, corn kernels are considered grains!) contain phytic acid, which is an anti-nutrient. Phytic acid binds with minerals like iron, zinc, calcium, and magnesium in the body, creating phytates that prevent the minerals from being absorbed properly. Without absorption, you can't reap the full benefits of these minerals.

These phytates can only be broken down by an enzyme called phytase, which releases the minerals and makes them available for absorption in the body. The problem is that there's very little phytase in the small intestine, which hinders the body's ability to digest phytates. This means that even if you're consuming enough minerals like iron, you may not be getting their full benefits. Interestingly, even though phytate may hinder mineral absorption, having undigested phytate in the colon may actually protect against colonic carcinoma.

Vitamin A (and beta-carotene, which converts to vitamin A in the body) can counteract the inhibitory effect of phytates on iron absorption. Vitamin A forms a complex with iron, which remains soluble in the intestine even at a pH of 6. This increases the availability of iron in the bloodstream for absorption.

Research indicates that normal levels of vitamin A (up to 900 µg) favor iron absorption. However, high doses of vitamin A (1800 µg) may lower iron absorption in the body. These high doses of vitamin A are generally possible with vitamin A supplements, not with foods. For best results, get these nutrients from natural food sources, not from vitamin supplements. Eat foods high in vitamin A, such as sweet potatoes, carrots, and pumpkin, with iron food sources such as beans, lentils, and spinach for maximum health benefits.

VITAMIN A + ZINC

Not having enough zinc in your diet can lead to a deficiency in vitamin A. To ensure you get the maximum health benefits of vitamin A, it's important to eat it with zinc-rich food sources. Zinc is crucial for all aspects of vitamin A metabolism, including absorption, transport, and utilization in the body. Without enough zinc, vitamin A (1) cannot be absorbed in the intestine (2) cannot be converted into retinal, therefore cannot be then converted to its active form (3) cannot be transported from blood circulation to body tissues, (4) cannot be released from its storage form, in the liver when needed. This limits the body's ability to use the vitamin A you consume. The combination of vitamin A and zinc also positively impacts your immunity, with vitamin A playing an important role in the production and function of white blood cells, and zinc is required for the development and function of cell-mediating innate immunity, natural killer cells, and neutrophils. Both nutrients also have antioxidant properties and help fight free radicals in the body. By eating them together, you can protect yourself against numerous chronic diseases.

To maximize the health benefits of vitamin A, eat foods rich in this nutrient, such as spinach, sweet potatoes, and red bell peppers, alongside zinc-rich options like chickpeas, kidney beans, cashews, pumpkin seeds, and oats.

VITAMIN E + SELENIUM

Research has shown that a combination of vitamin E and selenium has a synergetic effect, making it more effective in protecting against prostate cancer and atherosclerosis compared to using either of these alone.

Selenium acts as both an immunomodulator and an antioxidant. It is even more powerful than vitamins E, C, and A in terms of its antioxidant properties.

Both vitamin E and selenium are antioxidants that play a crucial role in protecting cells. They safeguard lipids, specifically polyunsaturated fatty acids, present in cell membranes from oxidative degradation caused by free radicals. If antioxidants do not shield these lipids, lipid peroxidation can occur, leading to the destruction of membrane lipids. This can be harmful to the viability of cells and tissues and can make you more susceptible to chronic diseases such as atherosclerosis, inflammatory bowel disease, asthma, Parkinson's disease, and kidney damage.

Both selenium and vitamin E are antioxidants, but they function differently. Selenium increases the reactivity of an enzyme called glutathione peroxidase (GPx), which helps protect the body from oxidative damage. On the other hand, vitamin E is a chain-breaking antioxidant that interrupts the chain reaction by pairing with free radicals and preventing them from pairing with lipids.

It is important to obtain selenium from your diet, as this mineral is highly potent in antioxidants but can also be highly toxic. To ensure a balanced intake, try incorporating vitamin E-rich foods such as almonds, peanuts, asparagus, spinach, and Swiss chard with selenium-rich foods like Brazil nuts, walnuts, sunflower seeds, chia seeds, flax seeds, broccoli, garlic, onion, cottage cheese, mushrooms, and brown rice.

UNIT 4

DIET PLAN

Here's a 10-day diet plan to include natural sources rich in vitamins A, D, E, and K in your diet. Repeat this diet plan every 10 days and you will never be deficient in fat-soluble vitamins.

Days	Fat-Soluble Vitamins (% Daily Value)			
	Vitamin A	Vitamin D	Vitamin E	Vitamin K
Day 1	1 baked sweet potato with skin (>100%)	Sunlight exposure for 30 minutes (>100%)	1 tablespoon wheat germ oil (>100%)	½ cup of cooked spinach (>100%)
Day 2	⅔ cup ice cream (20%) + 1 large cooked	1 cup UV-exposed cooked mushrooms with	A handful of dry roasted hazelnuts (30%) + 1	1 cup cooked okra (30%) + 1 cup pomegrana

	red bell pepper (15%) + 1 cup carrot juice (>65%)	cheddar cheese + + 2 tablespoons of butter	medium Kiwi (10%) + 2 tablespoons of safflower oil (60%)	te juice (20%) + 1 medium carrot (10%) + ½ cup roasted soybeans (40%)
Day 3	2 slices of papaya (20%) + ½ cup raw carrots (50%) + 1 cup vanilla ice-cream (30%)	1 cup soy, almond, or oat milk (20%) + 2 tablespoons of butter (2%) + 15 minutes of direct sunlight exposure	2 tablespoons of peanut butter (20%) + A handful of dry roasted hazelnuts (30%) + 1 cup cooked spinach (30%) + 2 medium kiwi (20%)	1 cup iceberg lettuce with Caesar salad dressing (25%) + ½ cup grapes (10%) + 1 cup cooked pumpkin (40%) + 100 g sprouted mung beans (25%)
Day 4	1 piece of pumpkin	Sunlight exposure for 20	2 tablespoons of	1 cup cooked soybeans

	pie (55%) + 2 slices of cantaloupe (25%)+ 2 mangoes (20%)	minutes + 1 cup milk with cereal (25%)	sunflower oil (80%) + 40 g of dry roasted peanuts (20%)	(80%) + ½ cup cooked edamame (20%)
Day 5	½ cup cooked spinach* (65%) + ½ cup raw carrots (50%)	UV exposed cooked white mushrooms 200 g (100%)	A handful of sunflower seeds and a handful of roasted almonds (95%) + 1 tomato	100 g cooked peas (25%) (*Spinach provides Vitamin A as well as Vitamin K)
Day 6	100 g cooked kale (55%) + 2 large mangoes (30%) + 30 g cheddar cheese (15%)	Sunlight exposure for 30 minutes	1 cup spinach cooked in 1½ tablespoons of sunflower oil (85%) + A handful of peanuts	1 cup cooked broccoli (>100%)

			(15%)	
Day 7	1 baked sweet potato with skin (>100%)	UV exposed cooked button mushrooms 200 g (>100%)	A handful of dry roasted sunflower seeds (45%) + ¾ cup broccoli cooked in 1 tablespoon of sunflower oil (55%)	½ cup cooked mustard greens (>100%)
Day 8	½ cup ricotta cheese (15%) + 1 cup milk (20%) + ½ cup cooked spinach (65%)	Sunlight exposure for 30 minutes (>100%)	1 tablespoon wheat germ oil (>100%)	½ cup cooked turnip greens (>100%)
Day 9	100 g pumpkin (55%) +	Sunlight exposure for 10	2 tablespoons corn oil	½ cup cooked collards

	2 slices of papaya (20%) + 1½ cup milk shake (25%)	minutes + other milk products such as yogurt, butter, cheese and milk powder	(30%) + 1 cup cooked spinach (30%), 1 large avocado (25%) +3 tomatoes (15%)	(>100%)
Day 10	100 g pumpkin (55%) + 2 slices of cantaloupe (25%) +1 cup milk** (20%)	Sunlight exposure for 20 minutes (**Milk contain Vitamin A and Vitamin D)	2 tablespoons peanut butter (20%)+ a handful of roasted almonds (45%)+ 2 kiwi (15%)	1 cup cooked broccoli (15%) + Vitamin K2 sources***

*** Vegetables and fruits provide vitamin K1, while milk and fermented foods provide vitamin K2, which is equally important. To get Vitamin K2, add curd, buttermilk, butter, cheddar, ricotta and cottage cheese, natto, idli, dosa, and dhokla (and other fermented foods) to your diet.

UNIT 5

RECIPES

Stir Fried Broccoli

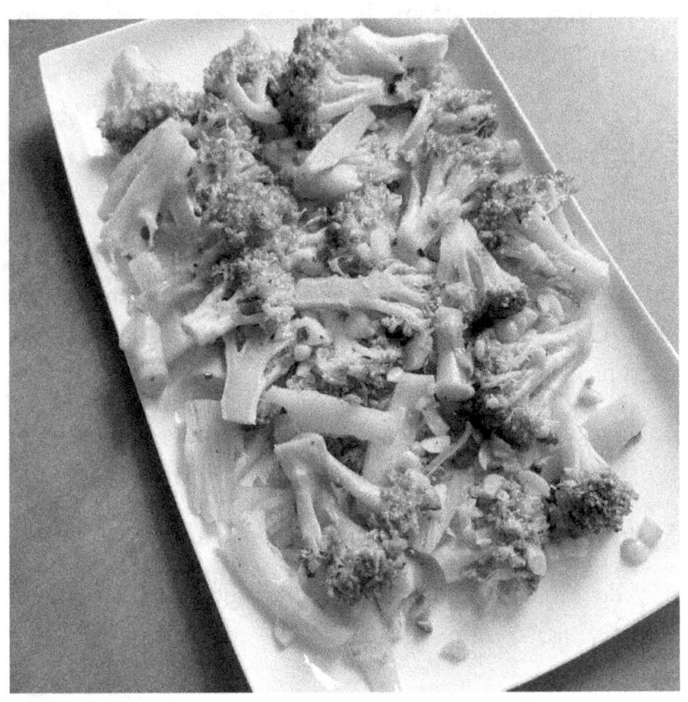

Ingredients

Broccoli: 1

Peanuts: 2 tbsp

Black pepper powder: ¼ tsp

Red chili flakes: a pinch

Garlic: 4 cloves

Asafetida: ¼ tsp

Salt: To taste

Sunflower oil: 1 tbsp

Method

1. Cut the broccoli into 1-inch pieces. Sprinkle salt on the broccoli and steam them in a steamer or pressure cooker, or para boil them in a saucepan.

2. Dry roast the peanuts in a hot pan until their color changes. Remove from heat and let them cool for a few minutes.

3. Place the roasted peanuts in a kitchen towel, cover them with a kitchen towel, and rub them to remove the skin. Crush the peanuts in a mortar and pestle or in a food processor.

4. Heat oil in a pan and add asafetida and chopped garlic to it. Cook them till they turn golden.

5. Add crushed peanuts and cook for 2 minutes.

6. Add broccoli, black pepper powder and chili flakes. Stir fry for 5 minutes and enjoy the crispy stir-fried broccoli.

Pan Fried Cheesy Mushrooms

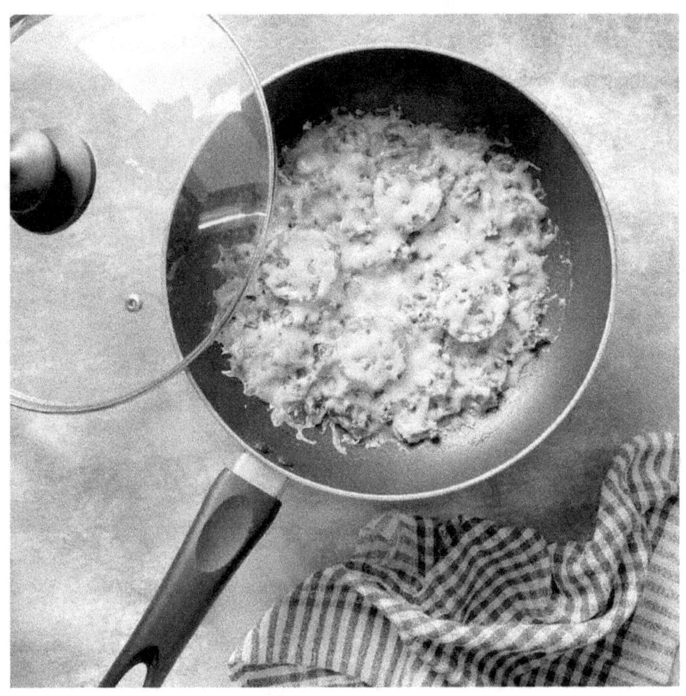

Ingredients

Button mushroom: 200 g	Cheddar cheese: 50 g
Cashew nuts: 30	Garlic: 5
Tomato: 1	Black pepper powder: ¼ tsp
Salt: To taste	Water: 100 ml
Butter: 1 tbsp	

Method

1. Wash and chop the mushrooms. Soak cashews in hot water for 2 hours. Grind them with water to make a thick paste.

2. Heat butter in a pan. Add chopped garlic to it and cook till it turns crisp. Take out the garlic from the pan.

3. Add chopped mushrooms, salt and black pepper powder. Cover and cook till all the water released by the mushrooms is re-absorbed.

4. Add cashew paste and mix well so that all the mushrooms get coated well in the paste. Cover with the lid and cook for 10 minutes. If it is sticking, then add 2 tbsp water.

5. Place tomato slices on top. Sprinkle salt and black pepper powder on the tomato slices. Cover and cook for 5 minutes till the tomatoes become soft.

6. Sprinkle fried garlic and shredded cheddar cheese over the mushrooms. Keep it covered for 2 minutes till the cheese melts.

7. Turn off the flame and enjoy piping hot Pan-Fried Cheesy Mushrooms.

Peas Avocado Soup

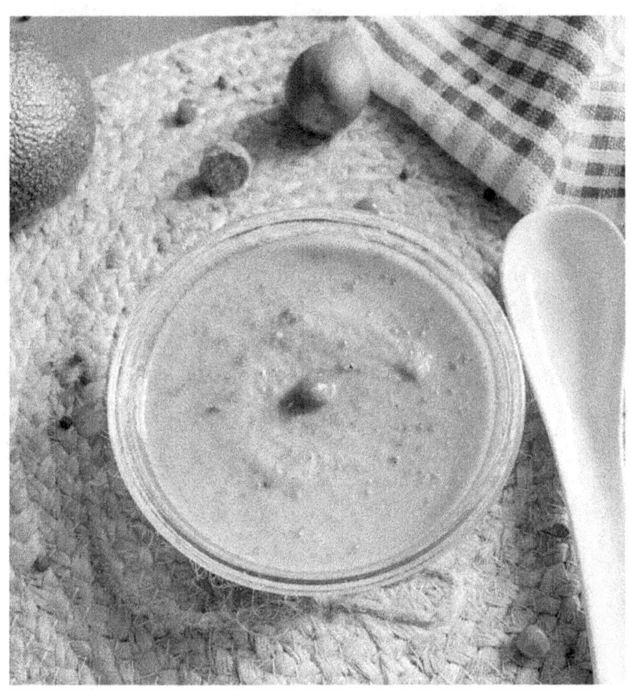

Ingredients

Avocado: 1 (170 g)

Peas: 100 g

White onion: 1 medium

Garlic: 5-6 cloves

Cumin seeds: ¼ tsp

Nutmeg: ½ small / ¼ tsp

Garam masala: a pinch / ¼ tsp

Black pepper powder: ¼ tsp

Curd: 2 tsp

Salt: To taste

Rice bran oil: 1 tbsp

Water 400 ml

Optional topping: ¼ tsp tandoori masala

Method

1. Heat oil in a saucepan. Add cumin seeds. When cumin starts crackling, add garlic and cook for 2 minutes.

2. Add chopped onion and cook till it turns slightly brown.

3. Add fresh peas and salt. Cover and cook till the peas become soft.

4. Lower the flame and add curd. Mix well and cook covered for 2 minutes.

5. Add a pinch of garam masala, black pepper powder and grate about half a small nutmeg. Cover and cook for 2 minutes.

6. Add 200 ml water. Cover and cook for 5 minutes till the water reduces slightly.

7. Add the remaining 200 ml water and cover again and cook for 5 minutes till the water reduces slightly.

8. Take a hand blender and blend the soup to make it thick and smooth.

9. Turn off the flame and add chopped avocado to it. Blend all the ingredients with a hand blender to make a creamy smooth pea avocado soup.

10. Take out the soup in a bowl and optionally sprinkle tandoori masala over it for a tangy taste.

Stuffed Bell Pepper

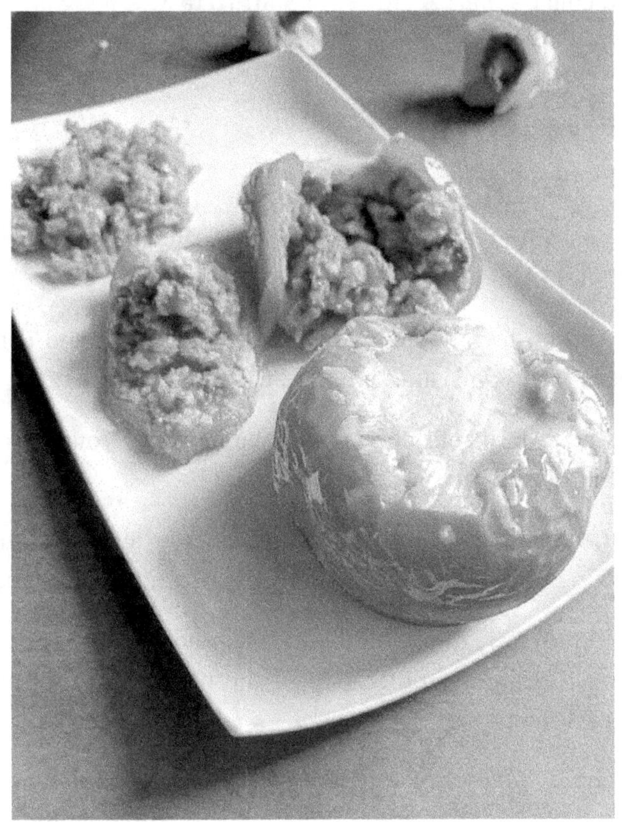

Ingredients

Red bell pepper: 4

Cheddar cheese: 100 g

Chopped onion: 50 g

Chopped cabbage: 50 g

Cottage cheese: 200 g

Chopped garlic: 2 tbsp

Chopped carrot: 50 g

Chopped green bell pepper: 50 g

Chopped pumpkin: 50 g   Chopped tomato: 50 g
Chopped mushroom: 50 g   Mixed herbs (oregano,
                          parsley, thyme): 1 tbsp
Red chili pepper: ½ tsp   Salt: To taste
Oil: 2 tbsp

Method

1. Preheat the oven to 190 °C.

2. Heat oil in a pan. Add chopped garlic and cook for 2 minutes. Add onion and cook for 5 minutes.

3. Add all the chopped vegetables one by one and cook until mushrooms and tomato release water.

4. Add salt, red chili pepper, mixed herbs (or your choice of herbs) and mix well.

5. Lastly, add crumbled cottage cheese and cook the stuffing until it becomes slightly dry. Turn off the flame.

6. Remove the tops of the peppers and scoop out the seeds. Grease the outer side of the pepper with oil and sprinkle some salt.

7. Grate some cheese inside the pepper and fill it with the prepared stuffing. Press the stuffing with the fingertip.

8. Place the bell peppers upside down in a baking tray and bake for 25 minutes at 190°C.

9. Remove the peppers and sprinkle a generous amount of cheese on top. Bake again, keeping the cheese side on top for 5 minutes until the cheese is melted.

Sarso ka Saag

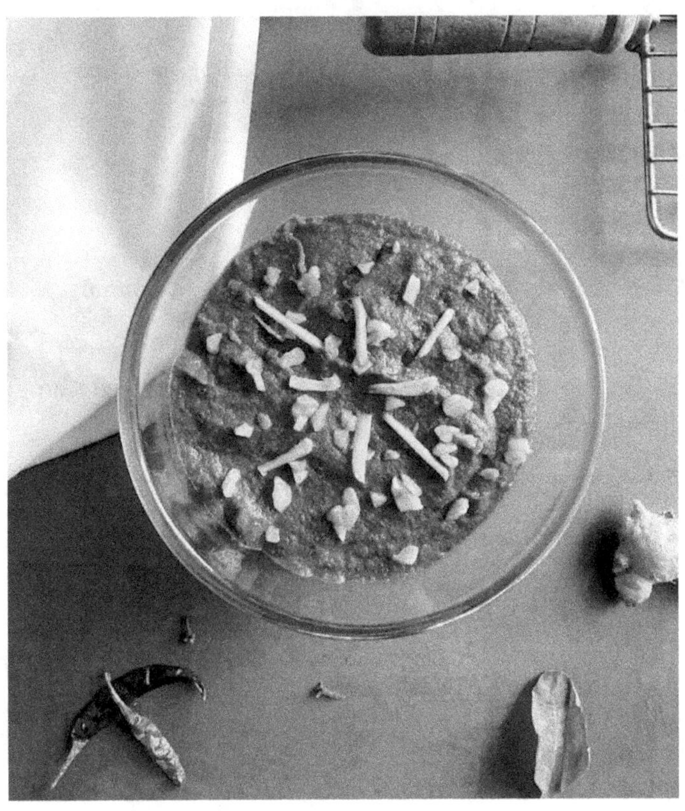

Ingredients

Mustard greens: 175 g

Spinach: 75 g

Lemon juice: 1 tbsp

Maize flour: 2 tbsp

Asafoetida: ¼ tsp

Cumin seeds: ½ tsp

Ginger: 1 inch

Garlic: 5 cloves

Onion: 3

Tomato: 1 medium

Garam masala: 1 tsp

Coriander powder: 1 tsp

Salt: To taste

Water: 250 ml

Rice bran oil: 2 tbsp

For Tampering

Ginger julienne: 1 tbsp

Chopped garlic: 1 tbsp

Asafoetida: A pinch

Red chilli: 1

Butter: 1 tsp

Method

1. Wash the mustard greens and spinach thoroughly. Cut them roughly.

2. Blanch the greens with 50 ml water, salt, and lemon juice for 5 minutes or till the greens are soft.

3. Let it cool down completely. Make a thick puree by grinding the greens with stock and green chilies.

4. Heat oil in a pan. Add asafoetida and cumin. Cook for one minute.

5. Add chopped ginger and garlic. Cook for 2-3 minutes.

6. Add chopped onions. Cover with a lid and cook on low flame for 10 minutes.

7. Add chopped tomatoes and salt (we have added salt during blanching, so add salt accordingly). Cover with a lid and cook on low flame for 10 minutes. Mash the tomatoes with a spatula.

8. Add garam masala and coriander powder. Mix well and cook for 5 minutes.

9. Add maize flour and mix well. Cook for 2 minutes. Add mustard greens and spinach puree and mix well.

10. Add 200 ml water and cook on low flame for 10 minutes. Keep stirring in between, and do not cover the greens. Turn off the flame and add tempering.

For Tempering

1. Heat butter in a pan and add asafoetida, ginger, garlic, and red chili to it. Cook the garlic till it turns brown.

2. Add this tempering to the prepared mustard greens. Immediately cover the greens with a lid. Keep aside for 10 minutes.

3. Enjoy Sarson ka Saag with makki ki roti (maize flour flatbread).

Tips:

1. You can also add other greens like chenopodium, collard, and radish greens with spinach. If using mixed greens, add 125 grams of mustard greens and 125 grams of mixed greens.

2. To retain the bright green color of the greens, do not cover them while blanching.

4. Very little salt is needed in sarson ka saag. You may need half or a quarter of the normal amount. So, add salt according to your taste.

Kiwi Smoothie

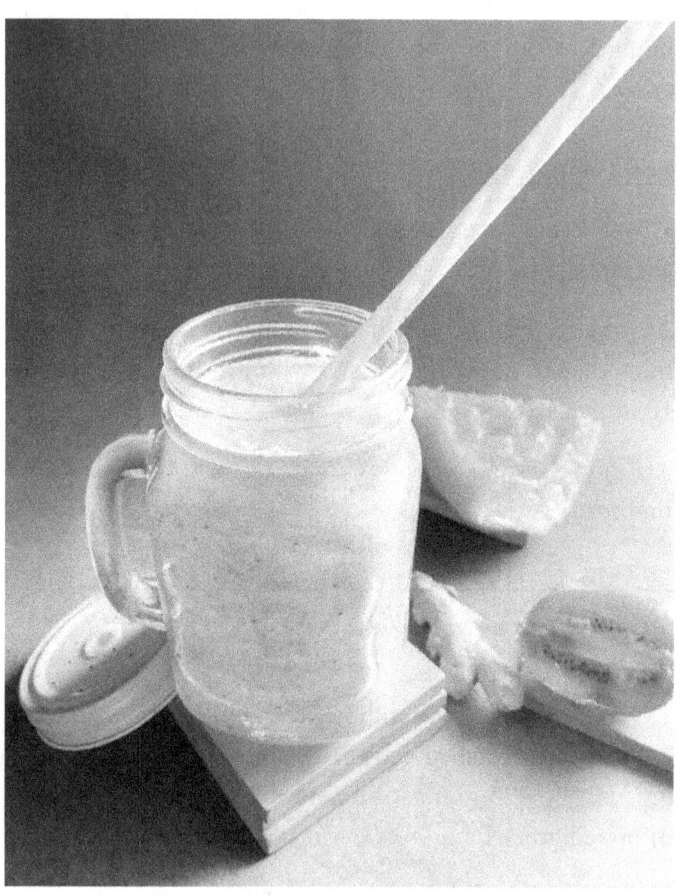

Ingredients

Kiwi: 2

Papaya: 150 g / 2 slices

Curd: 100 g

Chia seeds: 1 tbsp

Ginger: ¼ inch

Black salt: To taste

Water/Coconut water: 100 ml

Method

1. Soak chia seeds in plain water or coconut water for 2 hours.

2. Add kiwi, curd, papaya and black salt in a blender jar. Grate ginger and blend everything to make a smoothie.

3. Lastly add chia seeds and blend one last time to make a smooth kiwi smoothie.

Almond Avocado Pudding

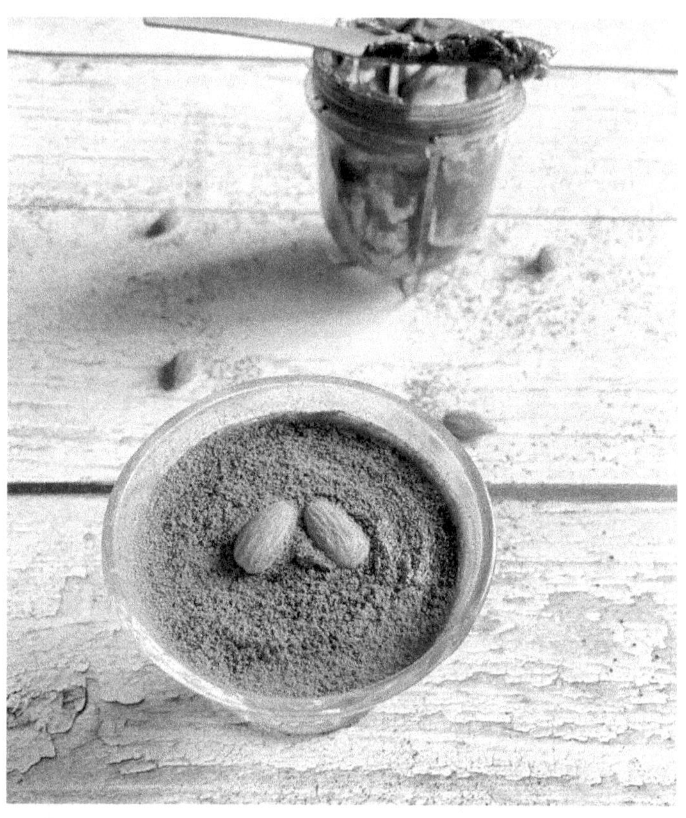

Ingredients

Almond: 50 gm

Avocado: 1 large

Cocoa powder: 2 tbsp

Honey: 2 tbsp

Extra virgin olive oil: 1 tbsp

Method

1. Dry roast the almonds in a hot pan till they change color slightly. Don't burn them; Otherwise, your pudding will taste bitter. Let the almonds cool down.

2. Blend the almonds in a food processor until they release oil. It will take some time, but eventually, it will turn into almond butter.

3. Add honey and extra virgin olive oil and blend again.

4. Add the chopped avocado to the jar and blend until the avocado is mixed with the almonds.

5. Lastly, add cocoa powder and blend to make a smooth, lump-free Almond Avocado Pudding.

The End

Sign up to La Fonceur Newsletter to receive Bonus Recipes:

https://eatsowhat.com/signup

READ PREVIOUS BOOKS OF THE EAT SO WHAT! SERIES

Book 1: Eat So What! Smart Ways to Stay Healthy

Book 2: Eat So What! The Power of Vegetarianism

REFERENCES

1. Albahrani AA, Greaves RF. Fat-Soluble Vitamins: Clinical Indications and Current Challenges for Chromatographic Measurement. Clin Biochem Rev. 2016 Feb;37(1):27-46. PMID: 27057076; PMCID: PMC4810759.
2. Multivitamin/Mineral Supplements Fact Sheet for Health Professionals, National Institutes of Health.
3. Conly JM, Stein K, Worobetz L, Rutledge-Harding S. The contribution of vitamin K2 (menaquinones) produced by the intestinal microflora to human nutritional requirements for vitamin K. Am J Gastroenterol 1994;89:915-23.
4. Suttie JW. Vitamin K. In: Ross AC, Caballero B, Cousins RJ, Tucker KL, Ziegler TR, eds. Modern Nutrition in Health and Disease. 11th ed. Baltimore, MD: Lippincott Williams & Wilkins; 2014:305-16.
5. Olorunnisola Olubukola Sinbad, Ajayi Ayodeji Folorunsho, Okeleji Lateef Olabisi, Oladipo Abimbola Ayoola, Emorioloye Johnson Temitope. Vitamins as Antioxidants. Journal of Food Science and Nutrition Research 2 (2019): 214-235.
6. Wiseman H. Vitamin D is a membrane antioxidant. Ability to inhibit iron-dependent lipid peroxidation in liposomes compared to cholesterol, ergosterol and tamoxifen and relevance to anticancer action. FEBS Lett 326 (1993): 285-288.
7. Vitamin and its importance. Drug Information Centre – Gujarat State Pharmacy Council.
8. Food fortification overview & regional update – World Health Organisation.
9. Guidelines on food fortification with micronutrients – World Health Organisation.
10. Datta M, Vitolins MZ. Food Fortification and Supplement Use-Are There Health Implications? Crit Rev Food Sci Nutr. 2016 Oct 2;56(13):2149-59. doi: 10.1080/10408398.2013.818527. PMID: 25036360; PMCID: PMC4692722.
11. Olson R, Gavin-Smith B, Ferraboschi C, Kraemer K. Food Fortification: The Advantages, Disadvantages and Lessons from Sight and Life Programs. Nutrients. 2021 Mar 29;13(4):1118. doi: 10.3390/nu13041118. PMID: 33805305; PMCID: PMC8066912.
12. Vitamin A and Carotenoids - Health Professional Fact Sheet - National Instiues of Health.
13. NUTRITION LANDSCAPE INFORMATION SYSTEM (NLiS) Nutrition and nutrition-related health and development data – World Health Organisation (WHO).
14. Huang Z, Liu Y, Qi G, Brand D, Zheng SG. Role of Vitamin A in the Immune System. J Clin Med. 2018 Sep 6;7(9):258. doi: 10.3390/jcm7090258. PMID: 30200565; PMCID: PMC6162863.
15. Clagett-Dame M, Knutson D. Vitamin A in reproduction and development. Nutrients. 2011 Apr;3(4):385-428. doi:

10.3390/nu3040385. Epub 2011 Mar 29. PMID: 22254103; PMCID: PMC3257687.

16. Capriello S, Stramazzo I, Bagaglini MF, Brusca N, Virili C, Centanni M. The relationship between thyroid disorders and Vitamin A.: A narrative minireview. Front Endocrinol (Lausanne). 2022 Oct 11;13:968215. doi: 10.3389/fendo.2022.968215. PMID: 36303869; PMCID: PMC9592814.

17. Zimmermann MB, Jooste PL, Mabapa NS, Schoeman S, Biebinger R, Mushaphi LF, Mbhenyane X. Vitamin A supplementation in iodine-deficient African children decreases thyrotropin stimulation of the thyroid and reduces the goiter rate. Am J Clin Nutr. 2007 Oct;86(4):1040-4. doi: 10.1093/ajcn/86.4.1040. PMID: 17921382.

18. Timoneda J, Rodríguez-Fernández L, Zaragozá R, Marín MP, Cabezuelo MT, Torres L, Viña JR, Barber T. Vitamin A Deficiency and the Lung. Nutrients. 2018 Aug 21;10(9):1132. doi: 10.3390/nu10091132. PMID: 30134568; PMCID: PMC6164133.

19. da Cunha MSB, Campos Hankins NA, Arruda SF. Effect of Vitamin A supplementation on iron status in humans: A systematic review and meta-analysis. Crit Rev Food Sci Nutr. 2019;59(11):1767-1781. doi: 10.1080/10408398.2018.1427552. Epub 2018 Feb 5. PMID: 29336593.

20. F.G. Huffman, Z.C. Shah. Encyclopedia of Food Sciences and Nutrition (Second Edition), 2003

21. Underwood BA. The Role of Vitamin A in child Growth, development and Survival. Adv Exp Med Biol. 1994;352:201-8. doi: 10.1007/978-1-4899-2575-6_16. PMID: 7832048.

22. Yee MMF, Chin KY, Ima-Nirwana S, Wong SK. Vitamin A and Bone Health: A Review on Current Evidence. Molecules. 2021 Mar 21;26(6):1757. doi: 10.3390/molecules26061757. PMID: 33801011; PMCID: PMC8003866.

23. Polcz ME, Barbul A. The Role of Vitamin A in Wound Healing. Nutr Clin Pract. 2019 Oct;34(5):695-700. doi: 10.1002/ncp.10376. Epub 2019 Aug 7. PMID: 31389093.

24. Elsa C Muñoz and others, Iron and zinc supplementation improves indicators of Vitamin A status of Mexican preschoolers, The American Journal of Clinical Nutrition, Volume 71, Issue 3, March 2000, Pages 789–794

25. Li Y, Wei CH, Xiao X, Green MH, Ross AC. Perturbed Vitamin A Status Induced by Iron Deficiency Is Corrected by Iron Repletion in Rats with Pre-existing Iron Deficiency. J Nutr. 2020 Jul 1;150(7):1989-1995. doi: 10.1093/jn/nxaa108. PMID: 32369598; PMCID: PMC7330461.

26. Hodge C, Taylor C. Vitamin A Deficiency. [Updated 2023 Jan 2]. In: StatPearls [Internet]. Treasure Island (FL): StatPearls Publishing; 2023 Jan-. Available from: https://www.ncbi.nlm.nih.gov/books/NBK567744/

27. Palace VP, Khaper N, Qin Q, Singal PK. Antioxidant potentials of Vitamin A and carotenoids and their relevance to heart disease. Free Radic Biol Med. 1999 Mar;26(5-6):746-61. doi: 10.1016/s0891-5849(98)00266-4. PMID: 10218665.

28. Murat Gürbüz, Şule Aktaç, Understanding the role of Vitamin A and its precursors in the immune system, Nutrition Clinique et Métabolisme, Volume 36, Issue 2, 2022, Pages 89-98, ISSN 0985-0562.

29. Carazo A, Macáková K, Matoušová K, Krčmová LK, Protti M, Mladěnka P. Vitamin A Update: Forms, Sources, Kinetics, Detection, Function, Deficiency, Therapeutic Use and Toxicity. Nutrients. 2021 May 18;13(5):1703. doi: 10.3390/nu13051703. PMID: 34069881; PMCID: PMC8157347.

30. Huang Z, Liu Y, Qi G, Brand D, Zheng SG. Role of Vitamin A in the Immune System. J Clin Med. 2018 Sep 6;7(9):258. doi: 10.3390/jcm7090258. PMID: 30200565; PMCID: PMC6162863.

31. Makita, T., Hernandez-Hoyas, G., Chen, T. H.-P., Wu, H., Rothenberg, E.V., and Sucov. A developmental transition in definitive erythropoiesis: erythropoietin expression is sequentially regulated by retinoic acid receptors and HNF4. H.M. (2001). Genes & Development, April 1, 2001.

32. Capriello S, Stramazzo I, Bagaglini MF, Brusca N, Virili C, Centanni M. The relationship between thyroid disorders and Vitamin A.: A narrative minireview. Front Endocrinol (Lausanne). 2022 Oct 11;13:968215. doi: 10.3389/fendo.2022.968215. PMID: 36303869; PMCID: PMC9592814.

33. Farhangi MA, Keshavarz SA, Eshraghian M, Ostadrahimi A, Saboor-Yaraghi AA. The effect of Vitamin A supplement on thyroid function in premenopausal women. J Am Coll Nutr. 2012 Aug;31(4):268-74. doi: 10.1080/07315724.2012.10720431. PMID: 23378454.

34. VanBuren CA, Everts HB. Vitamin A in Skin and Hair: An Update. Nutrients. 2022 Jul 19;14(14):2952. doi: 10.3390/nu14142952. PMID: 35889909; PMCID: PMC9324272.

35. Pozniakov SP. Mechanism of action of Vitamin A on cell differentiation and function]. Ontogenez. 1986 Nov-Dec;17(6):578-86. Russian. PMID: 3547226.

36. Shoya Iwanami, Shingo Iwami. Encyclopedia of Bioinformatics and Computational Biology, 2019

37. Clagett-Dame M, Knutson D. Vitamin A in reproduction and development. Nutrients. 2011 Apr;3(4):385-428. doi: 10.3390/nu3040385. Epub 2011 Mar 29. PMID: 22254103; PMCID: PMC3257687.

38. Pavlović, Dragan & Markišić, Merdin & Pavlović, Aleksandra & Lačković, Maja & Bozic, Marija. (2014). Vitamin A and the nervous system. Archives of Biological Sciences. 66. 1585-1590. 10.2298/ABS1404585P.

39. Sajovic J, Meglič A, Glavač D, Markelj Š, Hawlina M, Fakin A. The Role of Vitamin A in Retinal Diseases. Int J Mol Sci. 2022 Jan 18;23(3):1014. doi: 10.3390/ijms23031014. PMID: 35162940; PMCID: PMC8835581.

40. Wilhelm Stahl, Helmut Sies. Chapter 20 - Nutritional protection against photooxidative stress in human skin and eye. Academic Press, 2020, Pages 389-40.

41. Kim JA, Jang JH, Lee SY. An Updated Comprehensive Review on Vitamin A and Carotenoids in Breast Cancer: Mechanisms, Genetics, Assessment, Current Evidence, and Future Clinical Implications. Nutrients. 2021 Sep 10;13(9):3162. doi: 10.3390/nu13093162. PMID: 34579037; PMCID: PMC8465379.

42. Khoo HE, Ng HS, Yap WS, Goh HJH, Yim HS. Nutrients for Prevention of Macular Degeneration and Eye-Related Diseases. Antioxidants (Basel). 2019 Apr 2;8(4):85. doi: 10.3390/antiox8040085. PMID: 30986936; PMCID: PMC6523787.

43. Ram Reifen. Vitamin A as an anti-inflammatory agent. Proceedings of the Nutrition Society (2002), 61, 397–400 DOI:10.1079/PNS2002172.

44. Kawata A, Murakami Y, Suzuki S, Fujisawa S. Anti-inflammatory Activity of β-Carotene, Lycopene and Tri-n-butylborane, a Scavenger of Reactive Oxygen Species. In Vivo. 2018 Mar-Apr;32(2):255-264. doi: 10.21873/invivo.11232. PMID: 29475907; PMCID: PMC5905192.

45. Cheng J, Balbuena E, Miller B, Eroglu A. The Role of β-Carotene in Colonic Inflammation and Intestinal Barrier Integrity. Front Nutr. 2021 Sep 27;8:723480. doi: 10.3389/fnut.2021.723480. PMID: 34646849; PMCID: PMC8502815.

46. Blaner WS, Shmarakov IO, Traber MG. Vitamin A and Vitamin E: Will the Real Antioxidant Please Stand Up? Annu Rev Nutr. 2021 Oct 11;41:105-131. doi: 10.1146/annurev-nutr-082018-124228. Epub 2021 Jun 11. PMID: 34115520.

47. Yakıncı, Ömer & Süntar, Ipek. (2022). Vitamin A. 10.1016/B978-0-12-819096-8.00064-1.

48. Christophe Antille, Christian Tran, Olivier Sorg, Pierre Carraux, Liliane Didierjean, Jean-Hilaire Saurat. Vitamin A Exerts a Photoprotective Action in Skin by Absorbing Ultraviolet B Radiation. Journal of Investigative Dermatology,Volume 121, Issue 5, 2003, Pages 1163-1167, ISSN 0022-202X.

49. Fiedor J, Burda K. Potential role of carotenoids as antioxidants in human health and disease. Nutrients. 2014 Jan 27;6(2):466-88. doi: 10.3390/nu6020466. PMID: 24473231; PMCID: PMC3942711.

50. Polcz ME, Barbul A. The Role of Vitamin A in Wound Healing. Nutr Clin Pract. 2019 Oct;34(5):695-700. doi: 10.1002/ncp.10376. Epub 2019 Aug 7. PMID: 31389093.

51. Debreceni B, Debreceni L. Role of vitamins in cardiovascular health and disease. Research Reports in Clinical Cardiology. 2014;5:283-295

52. Zasada M, Budzisz E. Retinoids: active molecules influencing skin structure formation in cosmetic and dermatological treatments. Postepy Dermatol Alergol. 2019 Aug;36(4):392-397. doi: 10.5114/ada.2019.87443. Epub 2019 Aug 30. PMID: 31616211; PMCID: PMC6791161.

53. Sweet potato, raw, unprepared (Includes foods for USDA's Food Distribution Program) - US Department of Agriculture - Agricultural Research Service.

54. Khoo HE, Azlan A, Tang ST, Lim SM. Anthocyanidins and anthocyanins: colored pigments as food, pharmaceutical ingredients, and the potential health benefits. Food Nutr Res. 2017 Aug 13;61(1):1361779. doi: 10.1080/16546628.2017.1361779. PMID: 28970777; PMCID: PMC5613902.

55. Wu K, Erdman JW Jr, Schwartz SJ, Platz EA, Leitzmann M, Clinton SK, DeGroff V, Willett WC, Giovannucci E. Plasma and dietary carotenoids, and the risk of prostate cancer: a nested case-control study.

Cancer Epidemiol Biomarkers Prev. 2004 Feb;13(2):260-9. doi: 10.1158/1055-9965.epi-03-0012. PMID: 14973107.

56. Kale raw - US Department of Agriculture - Agricultural Research Service.

57. Peppers sweet red raw - US DEPARTMENT OF AGRICULTURE Agricultural Research Service.

58. Pumpkin, raw - US DEPARTMENT OF AGRICULTURE Agricultural Research Service.

59. Vitamin D Fact Sheet for Health Professionals, National Institutes of Health, Office of Dietary Supplements .

60. 25-hydroxy vitamin D test - MedlinePlus - National Library of Medicine.

61. Oliveri, Maria Beatriz, Mastaglia, Silvina Rosana; Mabel, et al.; Vitamin D3 seems more appropriate than D2 to sustain adequate levels of 25OHD: a pharmacokinetic approach; Nature Publishing Group; European Journal of Clinical Nutrition; 69; 6; 3-2015; 697-702

62. Wakeman M. A Review of the Potential Impact of Medication on Vitamin D Status. Risk Manag Health Policy. 2021 Aug 14;14:3357-3381. doi: 10.2147/RMHP.S316897. PMID: 34421316; PMCID: PMC8373308.

63. Sahay M, Sahay R. Rickets-vitamin D deficiency and dependency. Indian J Endocrinol Metab. 2012 Mar;16(2):164-76. doi: 10.4103/2230-8210.93732. PMID: 22470851; PMCID: PMC3313732.

64. Laird E, Ward M, McSorley E, Strain JJ, Wallace J. Vitamin D and bone health: potential mechanisms. Nutrients. 2010 Jul;2(7):693-724. doi: 10.3390/nu2070693. Epub 2010 Jul 5. PMID: 22254049; PMCID: PMC3257679.

65. Bener A, Ehlayel MS, Bener HZ, Hamid Q. The impact of Vitamin D deficiency on asthma, allergic rhinitis and wheezing in children: An emerging public health problem. J Family Community Med. 2014 Sep;21(3):154-61. doi: 10.4103/2230-8229.142967. PMID: 25374465; PMCID: PMC4214003.

66. Jat KR, Khairwa A. Vitamin D and asthma in children: A systematic review and meta-analysis of observational studies. Lung India. 2017 Jul-Aug;34(4):355-363. doi: 10.4103/0970-2113.209227. PMID: 28671167; PMCID: PMC5504893.

67. Sultan S, Taimuri U, Basnan SA, Ai-Orabi WK, Awadallah A, Almowald F, Hazazi A. Low Vitamin D and Its Association with Cognitive Impairment and Dementia. J Aging Res. 2020 Apr 30;2020:6097820. doi: 10.1155/2020/6097820. PMID: 32399297; PMCID: PMC7210535.

68. Yang CY, Leung PS, Adamopoulos IE, Gershwin ME. The implication of vitamin D and autoimmunity: a comprehensive review. Clin Rev Allergy Immunol. 2013 Oct;45(2):217-26. doi: 10.1007/s12016-013-8361-3. PMID: 23359064; PMCID: PMC6047889.

69. Gupta D, Vashi PG, Trukova K, Lis CG, Lammersfeld CA. Prevalence of serum vitamin D deficiency and insufficiency in cancer: Review of the epidemiological literature. Exp Ther Med. 2011 Mar;2(2):181-193. doi: 10.3892/etm.2011.205. Epub 2011 Jan 20. PMID: 22977487; PMCID: PMC3440651.

70. Vitamin D Fact Sheet for Health Professionals, National Institutes of Health.

71. Akimbekov NS, Digel I, Sherelkhan DK, Razzaque MS. Vitamin D and Phosphate Interactions in Health and Disease. Adv Exp Med Biol. 2022;1362:37-46. doi: 10.1007/978-3-030-91623-7_5. PMID: 35288871.

72. Fleet JC. The role of vitamin D in the endocrinology controlling calcium homeostasis. Mol Cell Endocrinol. 2017 Sep 15;453:36-45. doi: 10.1016/j.mce.2017.04.008. Epub 2017 Apr 9. PMID: 28400273; PMCID: PMC5529228.

73. Jacquillet G, Unwin RJ. Physiological regulation of phosphate by vitamin D, parathyroid hormone (PTH) and phosphate (Pi). Pflugers Arch. 2019 Jan;471(1):83-98. doi: 10.1007/s00424-018-2231-z. Epub 2018 Nov 5. PMID: 30393837; PMCID: PMC6326012.

74. Veldurthy V, Wei R, Oz L, Dhawan P, Jeon YH, Christakos S. Vitamin D, calcium homeostasis and aging. Bone Res. 2016 Oct 18;4:16041. doi: 10.1038/boneres.2016.41. PMID: 27790378; PMCID: PMC5068478.

75. Laird E, Ward M, McSorley E, Strain JJ, Wallace J. Vitamin D and bone health: potential mechanisms. Nutrients. 2010 Jul;2(7):693-724. doi: 10.3390/nu2070693. Epub 2010 Jul 5. PMID: 22254049; PMCID: PMC3257679.

76. Rak K, Bronkowska M. Immunomodulatory Effect of Vitamin D and Its Potential Role in the Prevention and Treatment of Type 1 Diabetes Mellitus-A Narrative Review. Molecules. 2018 Dec 24;24(1):53. doi: 10.3390/molecules24010053. PMID: 30586887; PMCID: PMC6337255.

77. Chen N, Wan Z, Han SF, Li BY, Zhang ZL, Qin LQ. Effect of vitamin D supplementation on the level of circulating high-sensitivity C-reactive protein: a meta-analysis of randomized controlled trials. Nutrients. 2014 Jun 10;6(6):2206-16. doi: 10.3390/nu6062206. PMID: 24918698; PMCID: PMC4073144.

78. AlJohri R, AlOkail M, Haq SH. Neuroprotective role of vitamin D in primary neuronal cortical culture. eNeurologicalSci. 2018 Dec 17;14:43-48. doi: 10.1016/j.ensci.2018.12.004. PMID: 30619951; PMCID: PMC6312860.

79. Wrzosek M, Łukaszkiewicz J, Wrzosek M, Jakubczyk A, Matsumoto H, Piątkiewicz P, Radziwoń-Zaleska M, Wojnar M, Nowicka G. Vitamin D and the central nervous system. Pharmacol Rep. 2013;65(2):271-8. doi: 10.1016/s1734-1140(13)71003-x. PMID: 23744412.

80. Prisant LM, Gujral JS, Mulloy AL. Hyperthyroidism: a secondary cause of isolated systolic hypertension. J Clin Hypertens (Greenwich). 2006 Aug;8(8):596-9. doi: 10.1111/j.1524-6175.2006.05180.x. PMID: 16896276; PMCID: PMC8109671.

81. Fisher SB, Perrier ND. Primary hyperparathyroidism and hypertension. Gland Surg. 2020 Feb;9(1):142-149. doi: 10.21037/gs.2019.10.21. PMID: 32206606; PMCID: PMC7082275.

82. Lips P, Eekhoff M, van Schoor N, Oosterwerff M, de Jongh R, Krul-Poel Y, Simsek S. Vitamin D and type 2 diabetes. J Steroid Biochem Mol Biol. 2017 Oct;173:280-285. doi: 10.1016/j.jsbmb.2016.11.021. Epub 2016 Dec 5. PMID: 27932304.

83. Palmer D. Vitamin D and the Development of Atopic Eczema. J Clin Med. 2015 May 20;4(5):1036-548. doi: 10.3390/jcm4051036. PMID: 26239464; PMCID: PMC4470215.

84. Abboud M. Vitamin D Supplementation and Sleep: A Systematic Review and Meta-Analysis of Intervention Studies. Nutrients. 2022 Mar 3;14(5):1076. doi: 10.3390/nu14051076. PMID: 35268051; PMCID: PMC8912284.

85. Laird E, Ward M, McSorley E, Strain JJ, Wallace J. Vitamin D and bone health: potential mechanisms. Nutrients. 2010 Jul;2(7):693-724. doi: 10.3390/nu2070693. Epub 2010 Jul 5. PMID: 22254049; PMCID: PMC3257679.

86. Krishnan AV, Trump DL, Johnson CS, Feldman D. The role of vitamin D in cancer prevention and treatment. Endocrinol Metab Clin North Am. 2010 Jun;39(2):401-18, table of contents. doi: 10.1016/j.ecl.2010.02.011. PMID: 20511060; PMCID: PMC5788175.

87. Vitamin D and Cancer, National Cancer Institute.

88. Garland CF, Garland FC, Gorham ED, Lipkin M, Newmark H, Mohr SB, Holick MF. The role of vitamin D in cancer prevention. Am J Public Health. 2006 Feb;96(2):252-61. doi: 10.2105/AJPH.2004.045260. Epub 2005 Dec 27. PMID: 16380576; PMCID: PMC1470481.

89. Vitamin E Health Professionals Fact Sheet, National Institutes of Health.

90. Kemnic TR, Coleman M. Vitamin E Deficiency. [Updated 2023 Jul 4]. In: StatPearls [Internet]. Treasure Island (FL): StatPearls Publishing; 2023 Jan.

91. Uchiyama K, Kishi H, Komatsu W, Nagao M, Ohhira S, Kobashi G. Lipid and Bile Acid Dysmetabolism in Crohn's Disease. J Immunol Res. 2018 Oct 1;2018:7270486. doi: 10.1155/2018/7270486. PMID: 30402511; PMCID: PMC6191959.

92. Vitamin E (Tocopherol) Test - MedlinePlus - National Library of Medicine.

93. Kretzer FL, Mehta RS, Johnson AT, Hunter DG, Brown ES, Hittner HM. Vitamin E protects against retinopathy of prematurity through action on spindle cells. Nature. 1984 Jun 28-Jul 4;309(5971):793-5. doi: 10.1038/309793a0. PMID: 6738695.

94. Effect of Vitamin E for Prevention of Retinopathy of Prematurity: A Randomized Clinical Trial.

95. Rosca MG, Vazquez EJ, Kern TS, Hoppel CL. Oxidation of fatty acids is source of increased mitochondrial reactive oxygen species production in kidney cortical tubules in early diabetes. Diabetes. 2012 Aug;61(8):2074-83. Epub 2012 May 14. PMID: 22586586; PMCID: PMC3402323.

96. Aprioku JS. Pharmacology of free radicals and the impact of reactive oxygen species on the testis. J Reprod Infertil. 2013 Oct;14(4):158-72. PMID: 24551570; PMCID: PMC3911811.

97. Bardaweel SK, Gul M, Alzweiri M, Ishaqat A, ALSalamat HA, Bashatwah RM. Reactive Oxygen Species: the Dual Role in Physiological and Pathological Conditions of the Human Body. Eurasian J Med. 2018 Oct;50(3):193-201. doi: 10.5152/eurasianjmed.2018.17397. PMID: 30515042; PMCID: PMC6263229.

98. S. Nazrun, M. Norazlina, M. Norliza, S. Ima Nirwana, "The Anti-Inflammatory Role of Vitamin E in Prevention of Osteoporosis", Advances in Pharmacological and Pharmaceutical Sciences, vol. 2012, Article ID 142702, 7 pages, 2012.

99. Zhang JM, An J. Cytokines, inflammation, and pain. Int Anesthesiol Clin. 2007 Spring;45(2):27-37. doi: 10.1097/AIA.0b013e318034194e. PMID: 17426506; PMCID: PMC2785020.

100. Konopatskaya O, Matthews SA, Harper MT, Gilio K, Cosemans JM, Williams CM, Navarro MN, Carter DA, Heemskerk JW, Leitges M, Cantrell D, Poole AW. Protein kinase C mediates platelet secretion and thrombus formation through protein kinase D2. Blood. 2011 Jul 14;118(2):416-24. doi: 10.1182/blood-2010-10-312199. Epub 2011 Apr 28. PMID: 21527521; PMCID: PMC4773892.

101. Kunisaki M, Umeda F, Inoguchi T, Nawata H. Vitamin E restores reduced prostacyclin synthesis in aortic endothelial cells cultured with a high concentration of glucose. Metabolism. 1992 Jun;41(6):613-21. doi: 10.1016/0026-0495(92)90053-d. PMID: 1640848.

102. Wu D, Liu L, Meydani M, Meydani SN. Effect of vitamin E on prostacyclin (PGI2) and prostaglandin (PG) E2 production by human aorta endothelial cells: mechanism of action. Ann N Y Acad Sci. 2004 Dec;1031:425-7. doi: 10.1196/annals.1331.063. PMID: 15753187.

103. Dayong Wu, Liping Liu, Mohsen Meydani, Simin Nikbin Meydani, Vitamin E Increases Production of Vasodilator Prostanoids in Human Aortic Endothelial Cells through Opposing Effects on Cyclooxygenase-2 and Phospholipase A2, The Journal of Nutrition, Volume 135, Issue 8, August 2005, Pages 1847–1853.

104. Lewis ED, Meydani SN, Wu D. Regulatory role of vitamin E in the immune system and inflammation. IUBMB Life. 2019 Apr;71(4):487-494. doi: 10.1002/iub.1976. Epub 2018 Nov 30. PMID: 30501009; PMCID: PMC7011499.

105. Cologne, Germany: Institute for Quality and Efficiency in Health Care (IQWiG); 2006-. What is an inflammation? 2010 Nov 23 [Updated 2018 Feb 22].

106. Lee GY, Han SN. The Role of Vitamin E in Immunity. Nutrients. 2018 Nov 1;10(11):1614. doi: 10.3390/nu10111614. PMID: 30388871; PMCID: PMC6266234.

107. Jiang T, Zhou C, Ren S. Role of IL-2 in cancer immunotherapy. Oncoimmunology. 2016 Apr 25;5(6):e1163462. doi: 10.1080/2162402X.2016.1163462. PMID: 27471638; PMCID: PMC4938354.

108. Coronary Heart Disease - National Health Service UK.

109. Waters DD, Alderman EL, Hsia J, Howard BV, Cobb FR, Rogers WJ, Ouyang P, Thompson P, Tardif JC, Higginson L, Bittner V, Steffes M, Gordon DJ, Proschan M, Younes N, Verter JI. Effects of hormone replacement therapy and antioxidant vitamin supplements on coronary atherosclerosis in postmenopausal women: a randomized controlled trial. JAMA. 2002 Nov 20;288(19):2432-40. doi: 10.1001/jama.288.19.2432. PMID: 12435256.

110. Lee IM, Cook NR, Gaziano JM, Gordon D, Ridker PM, Manson JE, Hennekens CH, Buring JE. Vitamin E in the primary prevention of

cardiovascular disease and cancer: the Women's Health Study: a randomized controlled trial. JAMA. 2005 Jul 6;294(1):56-65. doi: 10.1001/jama.294.1.56. PMID: 15998891.

111. Sesso HD, Buring JE, Christen WG, Kurth T, Belanger C, MacFadyen J, Bubes V, Manson JE, Glynn RJ, Gaziano JM. Vitamins E and C in the prevention of cardiovascular disease in men: the Physicians' Health Study II randomized controlled trial. JAMA. 2008 Nov 12;300(18):2123-33. doi: 10.1001/jama.2008.600. Epub 2008 Nov 9. PMID: 18997197; PMCID: PMC2586922.

112. Alkhenizan A, Hafez K. The role of vitamin E in the prevention of cancer: a meta-analysis of randomized controlled trials. Ann Saudi Med. 2007 Nov-Dec;27(6):409-14. doi: 10.5144/0256-4947.2007.409. PMID: 18059122; PMCID: PMC6074169.

113. Scanlan RA. Formation and occurrence of nitrosamines in food. Cancer Res. 1983 May;43(5 Suppl):2435s-2440s. PMID: 6831466.

114. Gugliandolo A, Mazzon E. Role of Vitamin E in Treatment of Alzheimer's Disease: Evidence from Animal Models. Int J Mol Sci. 2017 Nov 23;18(12):2504. doi: 10.3390/ijms18122504. PMID: 29168797; PMCID: PMC5751107.

115. Zhang SM, Hernan MA, Chen H, Spiegelman D, Willett WC, Ascherio A. Intakes of vitamins E and C, carotenoids, vitamin supplements, and PD risk. Neurology. 2002;59:1161-9.

116. Keen MA, Hassan I. Vitamin E in dermatology. Indian Dermatol Online J. 2016 Jul-Aug;7(4):311-5. doi: 10.4103/2229-5178.185494. PMID: 27559512; PMCID: PMC4976416.

117. Cook-Mills JM, Avila PC. Vitamin E and D regulation of allergic asthma immunopathogenesis. Int Immunopharmacol. 2014 Nov;23(1):364-72. doi: 10.1016/j.intimp.2014.08.007. Epub 2014 Aug 29. PMID: 25175918; PMCID: PMC4254328.

118. Dadkhah H, Ebrahimi E, Fathizadeh N. Evaluating the effects of vitamin D and vitamin E supplement on premenstrual syndrome: A randomized, double-blind, controlled trial. Iran J Nurs Midwifery Res. 2016 Mar-Apr;21(2):159-64. doi: 10.4103/1735-9066.178237. PMID: 27095989; PMCID: PMC4815371.

119. Koh ES, Kim SJ, Yoon HE, Chung JH, Chung S, Park CW, Chang YS, Shin SJ. Association of blood manganese level with diabetes and renal dysfunction: a cross-sectional study of the Korean general population. BMC Endocr Disord. 2014 Mar 8;14:24. doi: 10.1186/1472-6823-14-24. PMID: 24606630; PMCID: PMC3973834.

120. Jandacek RJ. Linoleic Acid: A Nutritional Quandary. Healthcare (Basel). 2017 May 20;5(2):25. doi: 10.3390/healthcare5020025. PMID: 28531128; PMCID: PMC5492028.

121. Oil, rice bran - US DEPARTMENT OF AGRICULTURE Agricultural Research Service.

122. Sheikh FS, Iyer RR. The effect of oil pulling with rice bran oil, sesame oil, and chlorhexidine mouth rinsing on halitosis among pregnant women: A comparative interventional study. Indian J Dent Res 2016;27:508-12.

123. Oil, cottonseed, salad or cooking - US Department of Agriculture. Agricultural Research Service.

124. Al Senaidy AM. Serum vitamin A and beta-carotene levels in children with asthma. J Asthma. 2009 Sep;46(7):699-702. doi: 10.1080/02770900903056195. PMID: 19728208.

125. Hwang JH, Lim SB. Antioxidant and anticancer activities of broccoli by-products from different cultivars and maturity stages at harvest. Prev Nutr Food Sci. 2015 Mar;20(1):8-14. doi: 10.3746/pnf.2015.20.1.8. Epub 2015 Mar 31. PMID: 25866744; PMCID: PMC4391535.

126. Wang T, Liu YY, Wang X, Yang N, Zhu HB, Zuo PP. Protective effects of octacosanol on 6-hydroxydopamine-induced Parkinsonism in rats via regulation of ProNGF and NGF signaling. Acta Pharmacol Sin. 2010 Jul;31(7):765-74. doi: 10.1038/aps.2010.69. Epub 2010 Jun 28. PMID: 20581854; PMCID: PMC4007727.

127. Lee S, Choi Y, Jeong HS, Lee J. Effect of cooking methods on the content of vitamins and true retention in selected vegetables. Food Sci Biotechnol. 2017 Dec 12;27(2):333-342. doi: 10.1007/s10068-017-0281-1. PMID: 30263756; PMCID: PMC6049644.

128. N. Kuppithayanant, P. Hosap and N. Chinnawong. The Effect of Heating on Vitamin E in Edible Palm Oil. International Journal of Environmental and Rural Development (2014) 5-2.

129. Guylaine, Ferland and James, Sadowski. Vitamin K1 (phylloquinone) content of edible oils: effects of heating and light exposure. Journal of Agricultural and Food Chemistry 1992 40 (10), 1869-1873. DOI: 10.1021/jf00022a028

130. Vitamin K - Health Professional Fact Sheet - National Institues of Health.

131. Widhalm JR, Ducluzeau AL, Buller NE, Elowsky CG, Olsen LJ, Basset GJ. Phylloquinone (vitamin K(1)) biosynthesis in plants: two peroxisomal thioesterases of Lactobacillales origin hydrolyze 1,4-dihydroxy-2-naphthoyl-CoA. Plant J. 2012 Jul;71(2):205-15. doi: 10.1111/j.1365-313X.2012.04972.x. Epub 2012 Jun 19. PMID: 22372525.

132. Beulens JW, Booth SL, van den Heuvel EG, Stoecklin E, Baka A, Vermeer C. The role of menaquinones (vitamin K_2) in human health. Br J Nutr. 2013 Oct;110(8):1357-68. doi: 10.1017/S0007114513001013. Epub 2013 Apr 16. PMID: 23590754.

133. Institute of Medicine (US) Panel on Micronutrients. Dietary Reference Intakes for Vitamin A, Vitamin K, Arsenic, Boron, Chromium, Copper, Iodine, Iron, Manganese, Molybdenum, Nickel, Silicon, Vanadium, and Zinc. Washington (DC): National Academies Press (US); 2001. 5, Vitamin K.

134. Shearer MJ, Fu X, Booth SL. Vitamin K nutrition, metabolism, and requirements: current concepts and future research. Adv Nutr 2012;3:182-95.

135. Ronald J. Sokol, Maret G. Traber. Vitamin E and Vitamin K Metabolism. Physiology of the Gastrointestinal Tract (Fourth Edition), 2006.

136. Vitamin K Deficiency Bleeding - Frequently Asked Questions (FAQ's): Vitamin K and the Vitamin K Shot Given at Birth - Centers for Disease Control and Prevention.

137. Lowenthal J, Birnbaum H. Vitamin K and coumarin anticoagulants: dependence of anticoagulant effect on inhibition of vitamin K transport. Science. 1969 Apr 11;164(3876):181-3. doi: 10.1126/science.164.3876.181. PMID: 5774189.

138. Shearer MJ, Newman P. Metabolism and cell biology of vitamin K. Thromb Haemost. 2008 Oct;100(4):530-47. PMID: 18841274.

139. The Emerging Role of Vitamin K2 Manouchehr Saljoughian, PharmD, PhD Department of Pharmacy, Alta Bates Summit Medical Center, Berkeley, California US Pharm. 2012;37(1):HS-12-HS-14.

140. Clinical and Research Information on Drug-Induced Liver Injury [Internet]. Bethesda (MD): National Institute of Diabetes and Digestive and Kidney Diseases; 2012-. Vitamin K. [Updated 2021 May 27].

141. Fu X, Harshman SG, Shen X, Haytowitz DB, Karl JP, Wolfe BE, Booth SL. Multiple Vitamin K Forms Exist in Dairy Foods. Curr Dev Nutr. 2017 Jun 1;1(6):e000638. doi: 10.3945/cdn.117.000638. PMID: 29955705; PMCID: PMC5998353.

142. Institute of Medicine. Dietary reference intakes for vitamin A, vitamin K, arsenic, boron, chromium, copper, iodine, iron, manganese, molybdenum, nickel, silicon, vanadium, and zinc. Washington, DC: National Academy Press; 2001.

143. Vitamin K Deficiency by Larry E. Johnson, MD, PhD, University of Arkansas for Medical Sciences - MSD Manual Professional Manual.

144. Goto S, Setoguchi S, Matsunaga K, Takata J. Overcoming the Photochemical Problem of Vitamin K in Topical Application. Vitamin K - Recent Topics on the Biology and Chemistry. IntechOpen; 2022.

145. Prothrombin Time Test and INR (PT/INR) - MedlinePlus - National Library of Medicine.

146. Shikdar S, Vashisht R, Bhattacharya PT. International Normalized Ratio (INR) [Updated 2023 May 1]. In: StatPearls [Internet]. Treasure Island (FL): StatPearls Publishing; 2023 Jan.

147. Cologne, Germany: Institute for Quality and Efficiency in Health Care (IQWiG); 2006-. What are blood thinners (anti-clotting medication) and how are they used? 2013 Nov 25 [Updated 2017 Oct 5].

148. Sørensen B, Tang M, Larsen OH, Laursen PN, Fenger-Eriksen C, Rea CJ. The role of fibrinogen: a new paradigm in the treatment of coagulopathic bleeding. Thromb Res. 2011;128 Suppl 1:S13-6. doi: 10.1016/S0049-3848(12)70004-X. PMID: 22221845.

149. Celia Rodríguez-Olleros Rodríguez, Manuel Díaz Curiel, "Vitamin K and Bone Health: A Review on the Effects of Vitamin K Deficiency and Supplementation and Effect of Non-Vitamin K Antagonist Oral Anticoagulants on Different Bone Parameters", Journal of Osteoporosis, vol. 2019, Article ID 2069176, 8 pages, 2019.

150. Maresz K. Proper Calcium Use: Vitamin K2 as a Promoter of Bone and Cardiovascular Health. Integr Med (Encinitas). 2015 Feb;14(1):34-9. PMID: 26770129; PMCID: PMC4566462.

151. Jamie Adams, Joseph Pepping. Vitamin K in Treatment and Prevention of Osteoporosis and Arterial Calcification. American Journal of Health-System Pharmacy. 2005;62(15):1574-1581.

152. Bügel S. Vitamin K and bone health. Proc Nutr Soc. 2003 Nov;62(4):839-43. doi: 10.1079/PNS2003305. PMID: 15018483.

153. Tsugawa, Naoko & Shiraki and Okano, T. Vitamin K status of healthy Japanese women: age-related vitamin K requirement for gamma-carboxylation of osteocalcin. Am J Clin Nutr 83: 380-386. The American journal of clinical nutrition. 83. 380-6. 10.1093/ajcn/83.2.380.

154. Ballegooijen AJ, Pilz S, Tomaschitz A, Grübler MR, Verheyen N. The Synergistic Interplay between Vitamins D and K for Bone and Cardiovascular Health: A Narrative Review. Int J Endocrinol. 2017;2017:7454376. doi: 10.1155/2017/7454376. Epub 2017 Sep 12. PMID: 29138634; PMCID: PMC5613455.

155. Li Y, Lu X, Yang B, Yasui T, Gao B: Vitamin K1 Inhibition of Renal Crystal Formation through Matrix Gla Protein in the Kidney. Kidney Blood Press Res 2019;44:1392-1403. doi: 10.1159/000503300

156. Girolami A, Ferrari S, Cosi E, Santarossa C, Randi ML. Vitamin K-Dependent Coagulation Factors That May be Responsible for Both Bleeding and Thrombosis (FII, FVII, and FIX). Clin Appl Thromb Hemost. 2018 Dec;24(9_suppl):42S-47S. doi: 10.1177/1076029618811109. Epub 2018 Nov 14. PMID: 30428703; PMCID: PMC6714837.

157. Xv F, Chen J, Duan, Li S. Research progress on the anticancer effects of vitamin K2. Oncol Lett. 2018 Jun;15(6):8926-8934. doi: 10.3892/ol.2018.8502. Epub 2018 Apr 16. PMID: 29805627; PMCID: PMC5958717.

158. Lu Xin, Ma Panpan, Kong Lingyu, Wang Xi, Wang Yaqi, Jiang Lingling. Vitamin K2 Inhibits Hepatocellular Carcinoma Proliferation by Binding to 17β-Hydroxysteroid Dehydrogenase. Frontiers in Oncology Vol 11 2021

159. Gary K. Schwartz, Manish A. Shah. Targeting the Cell Cycle: A New Approach to Cancer Therapy. Journal of Clinical Oncology 2005. PG 9408-9421. PMID - 16361640

160. Office of the Surgeon General (US). Bone Health and Osteoporosis: A Report of the Surgeon General. Rockville (MD): Office of the Surgeon General (US); 2004. 2, The Basics of Bone in Health and Disease.

161. Weber P. Vitamin K and bone health. Nutrition. 2001 Oct;17(10):880-7. doi: 10.1016/0899-9007(01)00709-2. Erratum in: Nutrition 2001 Nov-Dec;17(11-12):1024. PMID: 11684396.

162. Popescu A, German M. Vitamin K2 Holds Promise for Alzheimer's Prevention and Treatment. Nutrients. 2021 Jun 27;13(7):2206. doi: 10.3390/nu13072206. PMID: 34199021; PMCID: PMC8308377.

163. Alisi L, Cao R, De Angelis C, Cafolla A, Caramia F, Cartocci G, Librando A, Fiorelli M. The Relationships Between Vitamin K and Cognition: A Review of Current Evidence. Front Neurol. 2019 Mar 19;10:239. doi: 10.3389/fneur.2019.00239. PMID: 30949117; PMCID: PMC6436180.

164. Dasgupta S, Ray SK. Diverse Biological Functions of Sphingolipids in the CNS: Ceramide and Sphingosine Regulate Myelination in Developing Brain but Stimulate Demyelination during Pathogenesis of Multiple Sclerosis. J Neurol Psychol. 2017 Dec;5(1):10.13188/2332-3469.1000035. doi: 10.13188/2332-3469.1000035. Epub 2017 Dec 23. PMID: 30338269; PMCID: PMC6190913.

165. Wishart DS, Feunang YD, Guo AC, Lo EJ, Wilson M. DrugBank 5.0: a major update to the DrugBank database for 2018. Nucleic Acids Res. 2017 Nov 8. doi: 10.1093/nar/gkx1037.

166. Keith DA, Gundberg CM, Japour A, Aronoff J, Alvarez N, Gallop PM. Vitamin K-dependent proteins and anticonvulsant medication. Clin Pharmacol Ther. 1983 Oct;34(4):529-32. doi: 10.1038/clpt.1983.209. PMID: 6604612.

167. Lawson KD, Middleton SJ, Hassall CD. Olestra, a nonabsorbed, noncaloric replacement for dietary fat: a review. Drug Metab Rev. 1997 Aug;29(3):651-703. doi: 10.3109/03602539709037594. PMID: 9262944.

168. Food Additives Permitted for Direct Addition to Food for Human Consumption; Olestra. A Rule by the Food and Drug Administration on 08/05/2003

169. Lee, S., Sung, J., Choi, Y., Kim, Y., Jeong, H.-S., & Lee, J. Analysis of Vitamin K1 in Commonly Consumed Foods in Korea. Journal of the Korean Society of Food Science and Nutrition. The Korean Society of Food Science and Nutrition. 2015, August 31.

170. Khatun H, Rahman A, Biswas M, Islam AU. Water-soluble Fraction of Abelmoschus esculentus L Interacts with Glucose and Metformin Hydrochloride and Alters Their Absorption Kinetics after Coadministration in Rats. ISRN Pharm. 2011;2011:260537. doi: 10.5402/2011/260537. Epub 2011 Sep 11. PMID: 22389848; PMCID: PMC3263724.

171. Hsiao-Han Lin, Pei-Shan Tsai, Su-Chen Fang, Jen-Fang Liu. Effect of Kiwi Consumption on Sleep Quality in Adults with Sleep Problems. Asia Pacific Journal of Clinical Nutrition. (2011 / 06 / 01), P169 - 174.

172. CFR - Code of Federal Regulations Title 21 - US Food & Drug Administration.

173. Mung beans, mature seeds, sprouted, raw. Food Data Central. US Food & Drug Administration.

174. Peas, green, raw. Food Data Central. US Food & Drug Administration.

175. Khatun H, Rahman A, Biswas M, Islam AU. Water-soluble Fraction of Abelmoschus esculentus L Interacts with Glucose and Metformin Hydrochloride and Alters Their Absorption Kinetics. ISRN Pharm. 2011;2011:260537. doi: 10.5402/2011/260537. Epub 2011 Sep 11. PMID: 22389848; PMCID: PMC3263724.

176. Traber MG. Vitamin E and K interactions--a 50-year-old problem. Nutr Rev. 2008 Nov;66(11):624-9. doi: 10.1111/j.1753-4887.2008.00123.x. PMID: 19019024.

177. Schwalfenberg GK. Vitamins K1 and K2: The Emerging Group of Vitamins Required for Human Health. J Nutr Metab. 2017;2017:6254836. doi: 10.1155/2017/6254836. Epub 2017 Jun 18. PMID: 28698808; PMCID: PMC5494092.

178. Podszun M, Frank J. Vitamin E-drug interactions: molecular basis and clinical relevance. Nutr Res Rev. 2014 Dec;27(2):215-31. Doi: 10.1017/S0954422414000146. Epub 2014 Sep 16. PMID: 25225959.

179. Kim JM, White RH. Effect of Vitamin E on the anticoagulant response to warfarin. Am J Cardiol. 1996 Mar 1;77(7):545-6. doi: 10.1016/s0002-9149(97)89357-5. PMID: 8629604.

180. Drug Interactions between vitamin E and Warfarin - Professional from Drugs.com; c1996-2018.

181. Fan Y, Adam TJ, McEwan R, Pakhomov SV, Melton GB, Zhang R. Detecting Signals of Interactions Between Warfarin and Dietary Supplements in Electronic Health Records. Stud Health Technol Inform. 2017;245:370-374. PMID: 29295118; PMCID: PMC5760175.

182. Reddy P, Edwards LR. Magnesium Supplementation in Vitamin D Deficiency. Am J Ther. 2019 Jan/Feb;26(1):e124-e132. doi: 10.1097/MJT.0000000000000538. PMID: 28471760.

183. Toribio RE, Kohn CW, Rourke KM, Levine AL, Rosol TJ. Effects of hypercalcemia on serum concentrations of magnesium, potassium, and phosphate and urinary excretion of electrolytes in horses. Am J Vet Res. 2007 May;68(5):543-54. doi: 10.2460/ajvr.68.5.543. PMID: 17472456.

184. Uwitonze AM, Razzaque MS. Role of Magnesium in Vitamin D Activation and Function. J Am Osteopath Assoc. 2018 Mar 1;118(3):181-189. doi: 10.7556/jaoa.2018.037. PMID: 29480918.

185. Deng X, Song Y, Manson JE, et al. Magnesium, vitamin D status and mortality: results from US National Health and Nutrition Examination Survey (NHANES) 2001 to 2006 and NHANES III. BMC Med. 2013 Aug 27;11:187.

186. Al Alawi AM, Majoni SW, Falhammar H. Magnesium and Human Health: Perspectives and Research Directions. Int J Endocrinol. 2018;2018:9041694.

187. Lips P. Interaction between vitamin D and calcium. Scand J Clin Lab Invest Suppl. 2012;243:60-4. doi: 10.3109/00365513.2012.681960. PMID: 22536764.

188. Khazai N, Judd SE, Tangpricha V. Calcium and vitamin D: skeletal and extraskeletal health. Curr Rheumatol Rep. 2008 Apr;10(2):110-7. doi: 10.1007/s11926-008-0020-y. PMID: 18460265; PMCID: PMC2669834.

189. Lanham-New SA. Importance of calcium, vitamin D and vitamin K for osteoporosis prevention and treatment. Proc Nutr Soc. 2008 May;67(2):163-76. doi: 10.1017/S0029665108007003. PMID: 18412990.

190. Saboori S, Djalali M, Nematipour E, Saboor-Yaraghi AA, Eshraghian MR, Ramezani A. Various Effects of Omega 3 and Omega 3 Plus Vitamin E Supplementations on Serum Glucose Level and Insulin Resistance in Patients with Coronary Artery Disease. Iran J Public Health. 2016 Nov;45(11):1465-1472. PMID: 28032064; PMCID: PMC5182255.

191. M. Sepidarkish, M. Morvaridzadeh, J. Heshmati. Effect of omega-3 fatty acid and vitamin E Co-Supplementation on lipid profile: a systematic review and meta-analysis. Diabetes Metab. Syndr. Clin. Res. Rev., 13 (2019), pp. 1649-1656

192. Lu, T.; Shen, Y.; Wang, J.H.; Xie, H.K.; Wang, Y.F.; Zhao, Q.; Zhou, D.-Y.; Shahidi, F. Improving oxidative stability of flaxseed oil with a mixture of antioxidants. J. Food Proc. Preserv. 2020, 44, e14355.

193. Floros S, Toskas A, Vareltzis P. Bioaccessibility, Oxidative Stability of Omega-3 Fatty Acids in Supplements, Sardines and Enriched Eggs Studied Using a Static In Vitro Gastrointestinal Model. Molecules. 2022

Jan 9;27(2):415. doi: 10.3390/molecules27020415. PMID: 35056730; PMCID: PMC8780033.

194. Bischoff-Ferrari HA, Willett WC, Manson JE, Dawson-Hughes B, Manz MG, Theiler R, Braendle K, Vellas B, Rizzoli R, Kressig RW, Staehelin HB, Da Silva JAP, Armbrecht G, Egli A, Kanis JA, Orav EJ, Gaengler S.

195. Bischoff-Ferrari HA, Willett WC, Manson JE, Gaengler S. Combined Vitamin D, Omega-3 Fatty Acids, a Simple Home Exercise Program May Reduce Cancer Risk Among Active Adults Aged 70 and Older: A Randomized Clinical Trial. Front Aging. 2022 Apr 25;3:852643. doi: 10.3389/fragi.2022.852643. PMID: 35821820; PMCID: PMC9261319.

196. Maresz K. Proper Calcium Use: Vitamin K2 as a Promoter of Bone and Cardiovascular Health. Integr Med (Encinitas). 2015 Feb;14(1):34-9. PMID: 26770129; PMCID: PMC4566462.

197. Hu, L., Li, D. et al. The combined effect of vitamin K and calcium on bone mineral density in humans: analysis of randomized controlled trials. J Orthop Surg Res 16, 592 (2021). https://doi.org/10.1186/s13018-021-02728-4

198. Maresz K. Proper Calcium Use: Vitamin K2 as a Promoter of Bone and Cardiovascular Health. Integr Med (Encinitas). 2015 Feb;14(1):34-9. PMID: 26770129; PMCID: PMC4566462.

199. Institute of Medicine (US) Committee on Military Nutrition Research. Military Strategies for Sustainment of Nutrition and Immune Function in the Field. Washington (DC): National Academies Press (US); 1999. 13, Vitamin E, Vitamin C, and Immune Response: Recent Advances.

200. Traber MG, Stevens JF. Vitamins C and E: beneficial effects from a mechanistic perspective. Free Radic Biol Med. 2011 Sep 1;51(5):1000-13. doi: 10.1016/j.freeradbiomed.2011.05.017. Epub 2011 May 25. PMID: 21664268; PMCID: PMC3156342.

201. X. Chen, Rhian M. Touyz, J.B Park. Schiffrin. Antioxidant Effects of Vitamins C and E Are Associated with Activation of Vascular NADPH Oxidase and Superoxide Dismutase in Stroke-Prone SHR. Originally published1 Sep 2001.

202. García-Casal MN, Layrisse M, Solano L, Barón MA, Arguello F, Llovera D, Leets I, Tropper E. Vitamin A and beta-carotene can improve nonheme iron absorption from rice, wheat and corn by humans. J Nutr. 1998 Mar;128(3):646-50. doi: 10.1093/jn/128.3.646. PMID: 9482776.

203. Gabriel F, Suen, Marchini JS, Dutra de Oliveira. High doses of vitamin A impair iron absorption. Nutrition and Dietary Supplements. 2012;4:61-65.

204. Iqbal TH, Lewis KO, Cooper BT. Phytase activity in the human and rat small intestine. Gut. 1994 Sep;35(9):1233-6. doi: 10.1136/gut.35.9.1233. PMID: 7959229; PMCID: PMC1375699.

205. Vitamin A and Iron Interactions - International Vitamin A Consultative Group (IVACG).

206. Christian P, West KP Jr. Interactions between zinc and vitamin A: an update. Am J Clin Nutr. 1998 Aug;68(2 Suppl):435S-441S. doi: 10.1093/ajcn/68.2.435S. PMID: 9701158.

207. Baraboĭ VA, Shestakova EN. Selen: biologicheskaia rol' i antioksidantnaia aktivnost' [Selenium: the biological role and

antioxidant activity]. Ukr Biokhim Zh (1999). 2004 Jan-Feb;76(1):23-32. Russian. PMID: 15909414.

208. Mylonas C, Kouretas D. Lipid peroxidation and tissue damage. In Vivo. 1999 May-Jun;13(3):295-309. PMID: 10459507.

209. Noaman E, Zahran AM, Kamal AM, Omran MF. Vitamin E and selenium administration as a modulator of antioxidant defense system: biochemical assessment and modification. Biol Trace Elem Res. 2002 Apr;86(1):55-64. doi: 10.1385/BTER:86:1:55. PMID: 12002660.

210. Reagan-Shaw S, Nihal M, Ahsan H, Mukhtar H, Ahmad N. Combination of vitamin E and selenium causes induction of apoptosis of human prostate cancer cells by enhancing Bax/Bcl-2 ratio. Prostate. 2008 Nov 1;68(15):1624-34. doi: 10.1002/pros.20824. PMID: 18668529; PMCID: PMC2583090.

211. Dawn C. Schwenke and Stephen R. Behr. Vitamin E Combined with Selenium Inhibits Atherosclerosis in Hypercholesterolemic Rabbits Independently of Effects on Plasma Cholesterol Concentrations Originally. 24 Aug 1998.

212. Tinggi U. Selenium: its role as antioxidant in human health. Environ Health Prev Med. 2008 Mar;13(2):102-8. doi: 10.1007/s12199-007-0019-4. Epub 2008 Feb 28. PMID: 19568888; PMCID: PMC2698273.

213. Omega 3 fatty acids fact sheet – Health Professional Fact Sheet. National Institutes of Health Office of Dietary Supplements.

214. Patrick RP, Ames BN. Vitamin D and the omega-3 fatty acids control serotonin synthesis and action, part 2: relevance for ADHD, bipolar disorder, schizophrenia, and impulsive behavior. FASEB J. 2015 Jun;29(6):2207-22. doi: 10.1096/fj.14-268342. Epub 2015 Feb 24. PMID: 25713056.

ABOUT THE AUTHOR

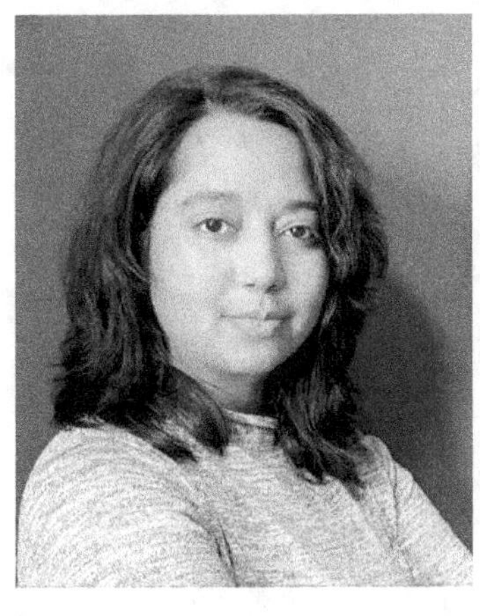

With a Master's Degree in Pharmacy, the author La Fonceur is a Research Scientist and Registered Pharmacist. She specialized in Pharmaceutical Technology and worked as a research scientist in the pharmaceutical research and development department. She is a health blogger and a dance artist. Her previous books include Eat to Prevent and Control Disease, Secret of Healthy Hair, and Eat So What! series. Being a research scientist, she has worked closely with drugs and based on her experience, she believes that one can prevent most of the diseases with nutritious vegetarian foods and a healthy lifestyle.

READ MORE FROM LA FONCEUR

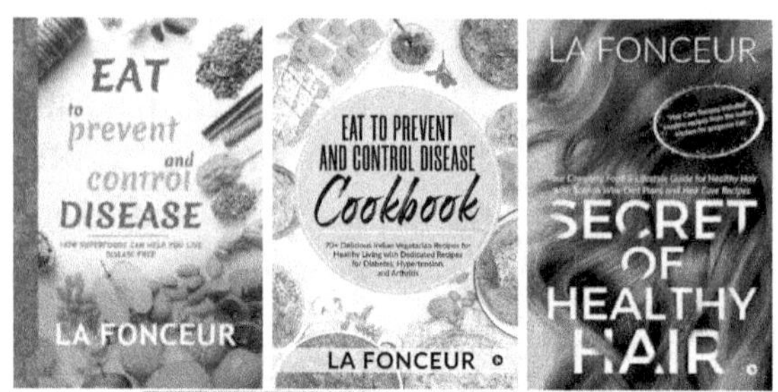

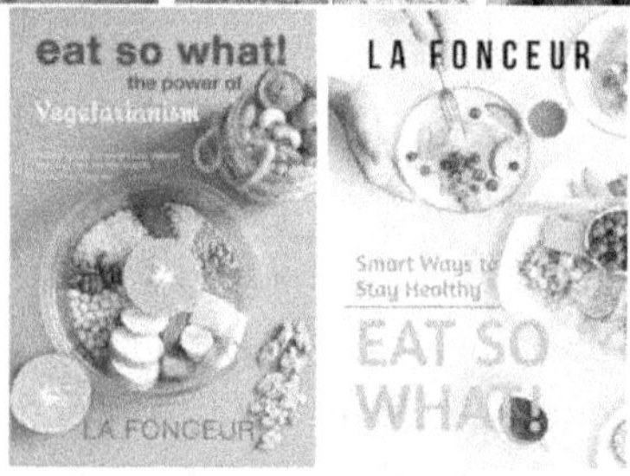

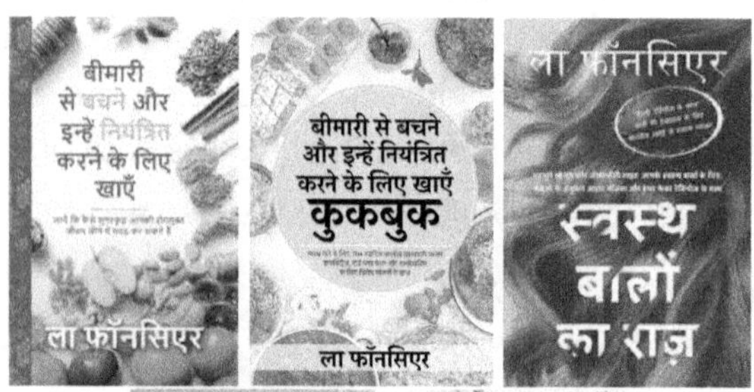

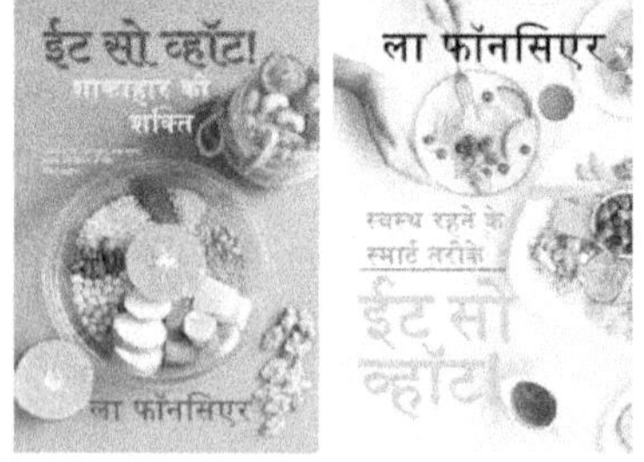

CONNECT WITH LA FONCEUR

Instagram: @la_fonceur | @eatsowhat

Facebook: LaFonceur | eatsowhatblog

Twitter: @la_fonceur

Follow on Bookbub: @eatsowhat

Sign up to get exclusive offers on La Fonceur books:

Blog: http://www.eatsowhat.com/

Website: http://www.lafonceurbooks.com/